SIMPLE, EFFECTIVE
TREATMENT OF AGORAPHOBIA

SIMPLE, EFFECTIVE TREATMENT OF AGORAPHOBIA

(previously published as
Agoraphobia: Simple, Effective Treatment)

Claire Weekes
M.B.E., M.B., D.Sc., F.R.A.C.P.

ANGUS & ROBERTSON PUBLISHERS

Unit 4, Eden Park, 31 Waterloo Road,
North Ryde, NSW, Australia 2113 and
16 Golden Square, London W1R 4BN,
United Kingdom

First published in Australia
by Angus & Robertson Publishers in 1977
First published in the United Kingdom by
Angus & Robertson (UK) in 1977
First paperback edition 1978
This edition 1983
Reprinted with corrections 1987, 1989

Copyright © Hazel Claire Weekes 1977

ISBN 0 207 14876 7 hardback
(not available in Australia)
ISBN 0 207 14877 5 paperback

Printed in Australia by
Australian Print Group, Maryborough, Victoria

8   7   6   5
94 93 92 91 90 89

While this book is for all medical therapists interested in treating agoraphobia and the anxiety state, I have been especially aware of the young general practitioner and the growing number of young para-medical workers in psychiatric and related medicine. These young people have rarely had the experience to match their special enthusiasm and dedication. I hope this book will give them such insight into their patients' most searching questions, that they will soon learn that satisfactorily answering such questions goes a long way toward curing the patients.

C.W.

Contents

Introduction

A therapist successful in treating the nervously ill is surely prepared to select from all available methods of treatment according to a patient's particular need. Dr Freud himself said that psychoanalysis failed to help some of his patients and that he was dejected when he saw them leave his care, still ill. Perhaps had he used a different approach to these people — even such as I describe in this book and which differs fundamentally from psychoanalysis — he might have been more successful with them. Unfortunately, some therapists are so dedicated and habituated to one method of treatment that they fail to appreciate the worth in others.

Talking about the success of our work rarely impresses unless supported by facts, so I will concentrate on presenting established facts: in 1972 I made a survey of 528 agoraphobic men and women in Great Britain, whom I had treated for periods ranging from one to seven years. The results of the survey, with emphasis on each patient's own estimation of his progress, were published in the *British Medical Journal,* 1973 and are included here pp. 4—10.

Many hundreds of thousands of copies of my first book[2] on nervous illness have been sold and the book is selling as well today as when first published in 1962. It has also been translated into eight languages. Also, hundreds of thousands of copies of my second book,[3] published in 1972, have been sold and it too has been translated into other languages.

The treatment described in the above works and in this book is followed today in many medical centres in Britain and the United States including phobic centres, psychiatric clinics and hospitals at some of which I have lectured on my visits to Britain and the United States during the last twenty years.

While the treatment appears simple, it is not easy and demands special understanding of the patient by the therapist. I have tried to give this special understanding here.

CLAIRE WEEKES

Sydney, 1987

Part 1: Understanding

CHAPTER ONE

Agoraphobia

In this book I am concerned mainly with the treatment of agoraphobia which, in my experience, is so often one phase of an anxiety state. The advice given can also be used in treating many people in an anxiety state uncomplicated by agoraphobia.

I have used this treatment over the last 40 years with gratifying results. It is now being adopted, particularly in Great Britain, by a growing number of psychiatrists, general practitioners and para-medical workers. For para-medical workers it has the advantage of not relying on any specialised aid; for example, it does not include electro-convulsive therapy, psychoanalysis, narcoanalysis, desensitisation according to current practice by behaviourists, or long-term medication.

The term agoraphobia derives from the Greek word *agora* meaning a place of assembly and the term phobia comes from the Greek *phobos* meaning flight, panic. The word agoraphobia was first used by Westphal in 1871 (Marks, 1969[1]). Dr Marks[1] says it is the most common phobia and represents 60% of phobic patients at the Maudsley Hospital, London. However, in my opinion, it differs fundamentally from monosymptomatic phobias such as fear of animals, germs and so on, and should not be classed with them. I discuss this later.

Agoraphobia is sometimes referred to as fear of open spaces. It could be more accurately defined as a condition in which a person suffers incapacitating fear away from the safety of home, particularly when in crowded or isolated places – anywhere where the sufferer cannot make quick escape or get help quickly should his fears, as he thinks, grow beyond him. It includes fear of travelling, especially in a vehicle he cannot stop at will.

In Great Britain during the last two decades, agoraphobia has been much in the news on radio, television, in newspapers and magazines. This interest has highlighted a pessimistic attitude toward its treatment and cure.* During Mental Health Week, 1974, a panel of psychiatrists on B.B.C. television concluded that the best treatment for agoraphobia was electroconvulsive therapy and/or drugs. I have never treated an agoraphobic patient with electroconvulsive therapy. In my opinion, electroconvulsive therapy is rarely a permanent cure for any anxiety state and in my patients agoraphobia has so often been one phase of an anxiety state.

Long-term treatment by drugs risks addiction, the appearance of side-effects, and robs a patient of confidence in a condition where the development of confidence is essential for recovery. A therapist surely admits defeat if he depends mainly on drugs for treatment of agoraphobia. It is not uncommon to hear an agoraphobic say, 'My doctor says I'll be on tablets for the rest of my life!' or, 'My doctor says agoraphobia can be controlled, never cured, and that I'll have to learn to live with it. He says I'll always have to take pills!' These two statements came from letters I received recently and over the years I have heard similar remarks from far too many agoraphobic people.

* During 1975, a move was made in the House of Commons to have agoraphobia rated as a handicapping illness.

After 40 years of practising, first as a general practitioner, then as a physician and finally as a consultant physician, with a special interest in the anxiety state (of which agoraphobia has so often been a part) and particularly after the last 24 years concerned almost exclusively with treating agoraphobic people not only in Australia but also in the United Kingdom and the United States, I consider that, from the results obtained, an optimistic approach to the treatment of agoraphobia is justified.

One of the reasons for pessimism among therapists is the difficulty in seeing agoraphobic patients often enough to give effective help. Part of an agoraphobic's illness is inability to travel alone (sometimes even if accompanied) to the doctor's surgery. Infrequent visiting is discouraging to both doctor and patient, especially during the early stages of recovery from agoraphobia when the patient needs special support and encouragement to help him through the setbacks that seem an inevitable part of recovery from this illness. To visit a patient often enough in his own home to meet these demands is surely asking too much from a busy therapist.

TREATMENT BY REMOTE DIRECTION

During 1966–74, I overcame the difficulty of visiting patients by treating (in addition to patients in private practice) approximately 2,000 agoraphobic men and women in Great Britain, Ireland, the United States, Canada, South Africa and Australia by remote direction in the form of two books [2,3], an album of two long-playing records[4], cassettes [5,6] for a small portable tape recorder and (1969–75) a quarterly magazine of direction and encouragement.

Treatment by remote direction has the advantage of offering help whenever a sufferer needs it (which may be many times in the one day) and where most needed, that is while trying to move from home when his symptoms, especially panic, are most severe. It also makes possible the treatment of people who live in places so isolated that they may not otherwise be able to get help. The books, records, cassettes and journals are available to any interested therapist (see references at end of book).

In 1970 I made a survey of 528 agoraphobic men and women in Great Britain and Ireland[7] whom I had treated by remote direction. Their ages ranged from 14 to 74 and treatment from one to seven years. The findings in the survey were so typical of the characteristics I have found among agoraphobic people in general that I include the most relevant facts here for future reference in this book.

Of the 528 patients concerned, 60% had been agoraphobic for 10 years or more and 27% for 20 years or more. so that most could be classified as chronic agoraphobics.

Sex. Some 91% were females.

Marital status. Of the 486 women only 51 were single; of 42 men, 16.

Occupation. Of the females, 78% were occupied by home duties, 12% by part-time work and 10% by full-time work away from home. Some 5% of the men were retired.

Present domestic conditions. Of those in their teens, twenties and thirties, 53% said they were happy, 45% unhappy and the remainder were passably happy. Of those in their forties, 56% were happy, 18% unhappy and 26% passably happy. In their fifties, 46% were happy, 8% unhappy, 46% passably happy. In their sixties, 41% were happy, 14% unhappy and 45% passably happy and in their seventies, 38% were happy and none was unhappy.

Conditions during childhood. Some 75% said their childhood was either very happy, happy or passably happy; only 25% had been unhappy.

Principal fears. The fears complained of were typical of agoraphobics in general: fear of being in crowded places, of travelling away from home either alone, or for some, even when accompanied, fear of 'collapsing', fainting, panicking, of feeling 'paralysed' in the street, giddiness, fear of entering shops, standing in a queue. Other less frequent fears were: being alone in the house, death, childbirth, physical illness, going mad, feelings of unreality, persistent frightening thoughts, fear of losing a loved one, harming others (especially a child), loss of confidence, depression, fear of accidents, insecurity, blushing. There were certain discrete phobias (such as fear of a specific animal) and obsessions (such as compulsive handwashing). Finally, some complained of a general anxiety without specific cause.

The most common fears amongst men were: fear of physical illness (especially coronary heart disease), of not being able to cope at work, insecurity, loneliness.

Cause of illness. Precipitating causes of agoraphobia given in order of frequency were: physical illness (for example, following a surgical operation, difficult confinement, tuberculosis, infection, arthritis), domestic stress in adult life, loss of loved one, difficulty or pressure at work, domineering parent or parents, a parent who had had a nervous breakdown (occasionally agoraphobia), unhappy parent or parents, an alcoholic parent, the sudden occurrence of frightening symptoms when out (for example, unexpected and hitherto unexperienced attacks of palpitations, giddiness panic), being an only child, having a nervous disposition, illegitimacy, the Second World War, strain of looking after an elderly parent or parents. Some 5% could give no cause for their illness and only 5 out of 528 people complained of sexual difficulties.

Age of onset of agoraphobia. The majority first became ill in their twenties or thirties. Dr Marks[1] wrote, 'It is not at all clear why agoraphobia should be a particular feature of young adult life, when people of all ages are exposed to the rigours of going into open spaces and streets. It is relevant that anxiety states have the same range of onset as the agoraphobic syndrome and that the two conditions overlap considerably in their clinical features, except that anxiety is mainly generalised, is not situational.'

When one sees agoraphobia arising so often in a patient in an anxiety state it is not difficult to understand how the range of its onset coincides with that of the anxiety state and since an anxiety state occurs most frequently in young people (particularly those in their twenties and thirties) it naturally follows that agoraphobia also occurs commonly in this age group. Also, 'going into open spaces and streets' is surely not a very rigorous undertaking unless one is already conditioned by an anxiety state into losing confidence in travelling alone, or in being in places where help cannot be quickly obtained.

The difference in sex incidence is also understandable because agoraphobia develops naturally in women whose work at home gives them opportunity to shelter there, if they so wish. Men working away from home must make the effort to leave the house daily and therefore do not so easily develop the agoraphobic syndrome. However, some men express their agoraphobia as a city-bound executive syndrome; that is, they avoid travelling to outer districts and other cities and may refuse promotion even if it means no more than occasionally travelling out of town.

Previous treatment. For their agoraphobia 65% had had treatment from one or more psychiatrists and 30% from a general practitioner only. The treatment given had included almost every known orthodox method: electro-convulsive therapy, psychoanalysis, narcoanalysis, hypnosis, behaviourism, modified leucotomy, insulin therapy, L.S.D., group therapy, occupational therapy and, in the words of many, 'drugs and more drugs'.

Results of previous treatment. Some 55% had received no help from previous treatment; 6% had been helped temporarily; 24% helped a little. Even those positively helped (15%) still needed additional help. These 528 people, therefore, offered a special challenge to any further treatment and particularly to treatment by remote direction.

Results of treatment by remote direction. Of the patients aged 14–29, the results were satisfactory or good in 73%; of those aged 30–39, similar results were found in 67%, and in those aged 40–49 in 55%. Of the older and therefore more difficult group aged 50–74, satisfactory or good progress was made in 49%. As so many of these 528 people were chronically ill (only 27 had been ill for less than three years) the chances of spontaneous recovery irrespective of treatment were negligible. By 'good' results I mean that these agoraphobics were able to move much more freely and if they panicked they could cope with the panic and were not especially deterred by it. Only 60 claimed cure; however, I learnt later that more considered they were cured but, as one man put it, 'To claim cure is too much like challenging fate!'

The following four examples are from the survey and are included to give the patient's opinion of satisfactory and good progress. Further examples are included at the end of this book.

SATISFACTORY PROGRESS
Male aged 61. Agoraphobic for 30 years 'on and off'. Cause: surgical operation followed by loss of job, plus war service, Second World War. Main symptoms: unreality, giddiness, fear of collapse, panic, inability to mix freely with people. Previous treatment: 'E.C.T. and various drugs. Three times as inpatient in hospital. It did not help me with the agoraphobia.' Treatment by remote direction, three years. Progress: 'With acceptance and self-desensitisation I have made more progress than over the last 20 years. I wonder if I am too late in starting for complete cure? I can now travel by bus alone on short journeys, stay alone in the house sometimes over the week-end when the others are away. Stand up to others instead of retreating. My doctor and friends say I look better.' Setbacks: 'These are my biggest problem. I feel well and then something occurs and I think I'm never to get completely cured; but now I keep on trying to occupy myself. It does pass. I have stopped spending money on so-called cures and with Dr Weekes's cassette I went on holiday alone this summer for the first time in years.'

SATISFACTORY PROGRESS
Female aged 51. Agoraphobic for ten years. Cause: 'In one year my father and brother both died, also my mother-in-law and father-in-law. My husband went into a mental hospital owing money everywhere and I lost all my

teeth; I felt quite defenceless.' Main symptoms: general anxiety, panic attacks when out and insomnia. Previous treatment: 'By general practitioner only for two years. He gave me drugs. They helped a little. My doctor is cynical about nervous illness, so it's no good going to him too often.'

Progress: 'I can now appear in public (bridge clubs, shops, hotels). Walk further than before and do my shopping fairly happily. My friends think I have improved. I get depressed by a setback but not for long.'

GOOD PROGRESS

Female aged 51. Agoraphobic for 19 years. Housebound. Cause: anaemia and domestic stress – full-time outside work and children to look after. Main symptoms: panic, jelly legs, blurred vision. Previous treatment: 'E.C.T., and drinamyl tablets for 20 years. Desensitisation at St Bartholomew's Hospital. It all helped a little.'

Progress with treatment by remote direction (seven years): 'I would say I am almost cured. I can shop alone in local shops; eat in a restaurant; walk to my daughter's about a mile away. I can do a door-to-door part-time job selling cosmetics; travel in public transport – buses, trams, underground! My daughters and friends say it is a miracle. I haven't had a setback since I started but still get the odd funny feelings. I try to float past them.'

GOOD PROGRESS

Male aged 43. Agoraphobic for six years. Cause: a 16-week period of illness starting with a slipped disc and followed by a virus infection which brought on an anxiety state. Main symptoms: fear of meeting people, panic, fear of setback. Previous treatment: 'Six years with general practitioner. It helped. Treatment was kindly encouragement and daily tablets.' Treatment by remote direction for four years.

Progress: 'First of all I understand how nerves trick you and also the part memory plays. This understanding gives me more confidence to treat myself when the first-fear starts. I am initially depressed when setback first strikes, but I reread the journals. Acceptance brings recovery.'

CHAPTER TWO

Sensitisation

The term 'desensitisation' is widely used today in psychiatry in conjunction with a modern method of treating phobias. Dr Marks[1] wrote, 'The method of exposing the subject to fear-producing stimuli may be important. One technique is to start with the stimuli exceedingly weak, distant, or remotely similar to the one feared and to approach the fear stimuli so gradually that only minimal fear is elicited and antagonistic responses can be applied. This is the method used in desensitisation.'

While the term 'desensitisation' is used frequently today, the term sensitisation is rarely used, and yet in my opinion it so often holds the key to understanding the development of both the anxiety state and agoraphobia. Dr Marks again wrote, 'We are left with the question of the origin of the general anxiety in agoraphobics. No one has yet answered this adequately.' In my opinion, to put agoraphobia in the first place and general anxiety in the second is to reverse their true order. The majority of my patients first developed an anxiety state from which agoraphobia arose as a secondary phase. In a few patients the anxiety state and the agoraphobia arose simultaneously.

By the term 'sensitisation' I mean a state in which emotional and nervous responses are greatly intensified and come with unusual, sometimes alarming, swiftness.

In a severely sensitised person nervous reactions to stress can be so swift he may think they come unbidden, as if (in words commonly used by patients) some 'thing' were doing this to him.

There is no mystery about sensitisation. Most of us have felt it mildly at the end of a day of tension when nerves feel on edge and trifles upset too much. Few are disturbed by mild sensitisation. On the other hand, severe sensitisation, such as the nervously ill person feels, can be most upsetting. A severely sensitised person feels the symptoms of stress so intensely that an ordinary spasm of fear may register as a whipping lash of panic, almost an electric flash, and is most bewildering because it can come in response to the slightest shock, no more than the unexpected slamming of a door, a sudden cold blast of wind, or more bewildering still, panic may flash for no apparent reason.

To understand agoraphobia one must above all appreciate the severity and swiftness of the panic that can come with sensitisation, and understand how, because of the ensuing fatigue and resensitisation, one flash of panic may quickly follow another, each flash mounting in intensity. Panic's alarming capacity to mount is one of the main reasons why an agoraphobic is reluctant to go where he thinks panic may strike.

I suggest that the physiological explanation of sensitisation lies in understanding how reverberated circuits in the nervous system work to produce a heightened response. The reverberated circuits in the autonomic nerves of the person in an anxiety state (which, as mentioned, so often includes agoraphobia) are usually initiated by fear, anxiety, dread, either as repeated stimuli or as sustained tension arising from a more or less constant background of stress. Through being so persistently alerted, nerves are in a more or less constant state of startle. The heightened responses of which the sensitised person complains are the usual symptoms of stress *greatly exaggerated* and, of these, panic spasms are the most sensitising, each spasm, as already mentioned, preparing the way for further and more intense spasms. In other words, the patient's recurring anxiety (reverberated circuits) produces physical nervous symptoms of increasing intensity (heightened response).

It is the intensity of these established nervous responses that prevents simple explanation of any deep-seated cause being enough to cure a sufferer, because so often the patient's recurring anxiety concerns the nervous symptoms themselves, especially the whipping lash of panic.

In this book I will use the term sensitisation to mean the exaggerated nervous sensations and the intense emotional responses found in many people in an anxiety state, as opposed to ordinary mild sensitisation which most people under stress experience from time to time.

The sensitised (and by this, I now mean intensely sensitised) person may complain of any of the following; a thumping heart, 'missed' heart beats, pain in the region of the heart, constantly quickly beating heart, attacks of palpitations, giddiness, sweating, agitation, tightness across the chest, a 'lump' in the throat, difficulty in swallowing solid food, a feeling of inability to take a deep breath, headache, extreme irritability, intestinal hurry, a feeling of fullness and burning in the face, easily induced weakness, blurred vision, aching muscles, and above all flashes of almost incapacitating panic and, if away from home, an almost overwhelming desire to escape to surroundings where he knows he will calm down and the panic will abate. These symptoms of acute stress originate mainly from stimulation of autonomic nerves (principally the sympathetic).

To the above symptoms of acute stress the effects of chronic stress may gradually be added: fatigue, apathy, retardation of thought and movement, loss of appetite, sleeplessness, depression. These symptoms are accompanied by marked vulnerability to the slightest added stress because of the exaggerated response from too easily startled autonomic nerves.

It is important for the therapist and the patient to recognise that an anxiety state may be not so much the expression of the mere presence of the symptoms of stress as of *their exaggeration in a sensitised body*.

An anxious person may worry continuously over some stressful problem and yet, despite stress symptoms, may work and function normally. It is not until continuous stress or the shock of some sudden overwhelming stress sensitises him and exaggerates the symptoms that he may become *concerned with the state he is in, perhaps even more concerned with it than with the original problem*.

Usually my agoraphobic patients became sensitised either (1) suddenly as a result of some shock to their nerves, such as a heavy haemorrhage, an accident, a difficult confinement, an exhausting surgical operation, or (2) more gradually as a result of debilitating illness, too strenuous dieting, living or working with a stressful life-situation and so on.

A woman debilitated after an exhausting surgical operation may find minor shocks, such as the slight impact of the cleaner's broom against her bed, shoot through her 'like a knife' and may find waiting (for example, simply for visitors to arrive) an almost unendurable strain – as if her nerves are physically stretched like tightly drawn wires that will snap if relief does not come quickly. She may be so upset by these experiences that she may lie in bed constantly worrying about them. There may be the added strain of apprehension about coping with the work at home should she return feeling like this. Any post-operative complication may bring added stress, and so more sensitisation, which may gradually change earlier spasms of fear into acute flashes of panic. The increasing severity of the panic brings further bewilderment, anxiety, so that other symptoms of stress may follow: racing heart, churning stomach and so on.

This woman is now in an anxiety state which may be aggravated by any difficult domestic situation she may meet on returning home. At this stage she may be so sensi-tised that she may, in the words of one woman, have only 'to think fear to feel fear'. It must be frightening to find that a mere flickering, anxious thought can be followed by a consuming flash of panic. The natural reaction is to become more anxious and so establish a cycle of sensitisation–fear–sensitisation. The way is now clear for the development of agoraphobia.

CHAPTER THREE

Development and Establishment of Agoraphobia

DEVELOPMENT

Agoraphobia, as we use the term today, differs fundamentally and significantly from monosymptomatic phobias such as fear of spiders, death, germs and so on. The person with a specific phobia is afraid of an object *outside himself* and he fears it for its own sake – its feel, look, potentialities. The agoraphobic fears certain situations but not in quite the same way. He fears the feelings that arise *within himself* – the panic, weakness, palpitations – when in such a situation. He fears having a 'turn' where he cannot get help quickly, or where he thinks he may make a spectacle of himself in front of others. It would be logical to find a new name for the condition just described and keep the term agoraphobia for the rare, uncomplicated fear of open spaces or the market place (crowded places) per se. However, the term agoraphobia is so widely used today, even by the patients, to embrace a syndrome of multiple fears and symptoms, that I will continue to use it here in this way.

Sensitisation may be present without necessarily leading to nervous illness; hence the necessity to differentiate between the two. We could say a person is nervously ill when sensitisation persists and upsets him enough to interfere with his way of life.

I use the term illness not in the sense that it is a disease but that sensitised nerves respond so swiftly, intensely, that their victim feels ill. I could use the term disturbed instead of ill, but I think the distinction unnecessary. In his book, *The Myth of Mental Illness,* Dr Thomas Szasz writes, 'To understand psychiatry we must also understand the concept of mental illness, which arises in part from the fact that it is possible for a person to act as if he were sick without actually having a bodily illness. Should we treat him as if he were not ill, or as if he were?' and again, 'I hold that psychiatric interventions are aimed at moral, not medical problems.'

Although my treatment of sensitisation is based on altering the mood of the patient's approach to his condition, I am aiming at curing *a definite upset in physical nervous functioning (heightened response)* which, for convenience, I shall continue to call nervous illness. Also, in this book I use the term nervous illness to mean the anxiety state, either with or without agoraphobia as an accompanying phase, as distinct from a psychosis.

Bewilderment and fear are the culprits that prolong sensitisation and keep it severe. Bewilderment acts by placing a sensitised person under the strain of repeatedly asking himself, 'What is happening to me? Why am I like this?' Since fighting is our natural defence, the sensitised person almost invariably tries to fight his way out of bewilderment back to being the person he was before this 'thing' happened to him. However, the more he struggles, the more stress he adds, especially when his efforts are accompanied by so much tension, and of course *the more stress he adds, the more sensitised he becomes.* Failure to find a way out of the maze of upsetting symptoms makes the sufferer feel incapable of coping, not only with any present difficulty (for example, stressful domestic problems) but also with whatever future suffering he imagines his illness may bring.

He is doubly anxious because, as already mentioned, he has only to think fear to feel fear. Indeed, in a sensitised person the connection between merely slightly anxious thought and intense panic may be so close that its victim may be unaware of the thought and may believe that panic has struck 'out-of-the-blue', and because panic can seem to overwhelm him before he has time to cope with it, he may be convinced that he cannot direct his own thoughts, actions. The stress of bewilderment and fear being continually added to sensitisation keeps nervous symptoms severe and so helps to keep the sufferer nervously ill.

Sensitisation, bewilderment and fear were the three main pitfalls leading the majority of my nervously ill patients into an anxiety state and hence, so often, into agoraphobia. To express this simply many sufferers were in a cycle of fear-adrenalin-fear. *The development of agoraphobia – fear of leaving the protection of home – was a logical sequence of this.*

The sufferer rarely recognises his symptoms as no more than exaggerated responses to stress, because exaggeration makes them so different from the ordinary mild stress symptoms he has experienced from time to time. He thinks his symptoms unique; that no one could have suffered this way before. Sometimes he is so frightened, bewildered, he thinks he must be going mad. To learn that his symptoms follow a well-known pattern and that others suffer as he does brings enough relief to cure some people. However, the sufferer may be given no adequate explanation of his symptoms and be left bewildered and afraid. Too many people who have had psychiatric treatment, sometimes for years, and from more than one therapist, say, 'I've never had my symptoms explained before. If only I'd been told that years ago!' By 'years ago' the speaker could mean 20 years or more, occasionally as many as 40 years.

One woman, in the 1970 survey, in answer to my question about the cause of her illness, wrote, 'I had been found unconscious in the street. I was taken to hospital where I was examined. Nothing abnormal was found. I was not questioned about what drugs I was taking, nor did I think to tell the doctor. I suffered from low blood pressure and was taking priscol for the circulation in my hands with the result that after I left hospital I continued to take the priscol and to have very vague feelings, which ended in my finally being afraid to go out.

'I saw a psychiatrist. After hearing my story he said that I was identifying myself with my mother, who had died of cancer which had affected her brain. I had nursed my mother. I was 21 at the time. I had an encephalogram. There was some doubt about a brain tumour. I was sent to a different hospital in a reserved compartment on the train with an ambulance to meet the train. I went through the same procedure at this hospital and was given a clean bill of health.

'I have been agoraphobic now for 17 years. If only someone had said on that fatal day when I first went to hospital, "You normally have a low blood pressure. Priscol lowers blood pressure. So, all that happened was that you had a further fall in blood pressure due to the priscol and this made you faint," I know I would never have had agoraphobia. I loved walking before that incident. During the war I walked miles alone at all hours of the night with never the slightest feeling of fear.'

In my 1970 survey, 60% of the agoraphobic men and women had been ill for some 10 years or more; 27% for 20 years or more. Some 95% of the 528 people had had previous treatment for their agoraphobia and 55% said they had gained no benefit from it; 24% had been helped only a little and 6% helped temporarily. Perhaps the key to these disappointing figures is the lack of adequate explanation of the illness to the sufferer and unfortunately this is too often due to lack of sufficient understanding amongst therapists themselves.

ORIGINAL CAUSES OF SENSITISATION

Most of the agoraphobics I have treated had no doubt about the original cause of their illness. Only 5·6% in the 1970 survey said they knew of no original cause. In my opinion, too much time is spent today and too much suffering is caused by searching for a deep-seated cause for an anxiety state and consequently any accompanying agoraphobia in people in whom no such cause exists.

Even when a deep-seated cause is found, cure does not necessarily follow its exposure. It is usually not enough to tell a patient that such and such happened when he was young and that that is the reason for his present illness. *Present sensitisation so often remains because the habit of fear has become important now. This must be cured.*

One woman wrote, 'I saw a doctor four years ago. Out of sheer frustration and continually rehashing the past, I quit. All I seemed to hear was that my mother didn't love me and left me to the maids and that my father didn't love me either. I have been told over and over again that lack of love caused my acute phobias, but never how to handle the fears themselves, especially the fear of leaving home alone. I have repeatedly asked for help to deal with the constant fears, with the awful physical sensations I have. It seems all I have been given to live with is "if only. . . !".' This is a typical story.

COMMON CAUSES OF AGORAPHOBIA

The most common precipitating causes of agoraphobia given by men and women in the 1970 survey were, in order of importance: physical illness, stress at home or at work, difficult confinement, a sudden unexpected attack of panic, palpitations or severe weakness while out, depression, sorrow. Only five of the 528 people mentioned sexual problems.

Physical illness far outnumbered the other causes. However, all causes shared the common denominator, *stress*, which led to the development of sensitisation and which sometimes first declared itself in the street as an attack of panic, palpitations or a feeling of collapse.

PANIC

Mistakes in judging the stability of agoraphobics arise mainly from not understanding the intensity of the panic brought by sensitisation. It can be the crack of the stockman's whip! Also, sensitised sympathetic nerves can be so easily startled that one flash of panic may follow the other like a chain reaction in almost paralysingly quick succession. Understanding the electrifying quality of sensitised panic is the key to understanding how fear of it can arise in people hitherto not given to panicking. Dr Marks[1] remarked that agoraphobics represent a cross-section of the community and are not especially neurotic. This has also been my experience with patients. Of course there are always hypochondriacs who panic easily at any physical mishap, and readily develop an anxiety state. They are soon recognised by a skilled therapist.

As sensitisation progresses, any emotional reaction, not only panic, may follow thought so quickly that emotion seems to dominate thought. The sufferer feels this reaction so intensely that he may say his mind goes numb at the peak of panic; hence his reluctance to go out alone or be anywhere where he feels trapped, hemmed in or isolated. This is why he sits near the aisle at the cinema, near the door at the restaurant, at the end of the pew at the back of the church – 'just in case!'.

The fear of being caught in this way was well demonstrated by one man who could stand in a queue at the bank comparatively calmly until the moment when the teller took his bankbook. He knew then that he was trapped until the book was returned. This kind of sufferer is terrified because he thinks his panic may reach such a climax that he will lose control of himself (he never quite knows how) and be taken away somewhere (he never quite knows where, but an asylum looms among the possibilities).

In my experience with agoraphobic patients, panic while out is the symptom above all others that keeps the sufferer prisoner in his own home.

PALPITATIONS

When palpitations or a feeling of collapse (or perhaps both) are the presenting symptoms, they are usually quickly followed by bewilderment and fear and then perhaps by other symptoms of stress – panic, giddiness – as the victim tries to hurry home or find some nearby refuge as quickly as possible.

Anything unusual to do with the heart is upsetting and an attack of palpitations can be alarming, especially if it comes where the sufferer cannot get help. If, during the days that follow, he has further attacks, he is soon convinced there is something radically wrong with his heart. If he accepts his doctor's assurance that there is not, all may be well. However, if he is not adequately reassured, he may become reluctant to move from home and may remain so anxious that the whole hierarchy of nervous symptoms may appear: quickly beating heart, sweating hands, churning stomach, and so on. If the sufferer is a woman, there may be no necessity for her to leave the house alone, and she may so consistently avoid doing so that she may become gradually entrenched at home and totally dependent on others for help to move out-of-doors. This reluctance may be further reinforced if, on plucking up courage and venturing out by herself, her apprehension brings on an attack of panic, possibly followed by palpitations. She soon becomes adept at making excuses to avoid leaving the house. I have known such women to cling to home for years leaving it only when absolutely unavoidable, and yet, so well have they hidden their fears, their families have been unaware of their disability.

As mentioned, a man is usually obliged to travel from home to work, hence, while it is estimated that as many men as women suffer from an anxiety state, relatively few men suffer from agoraphobia; in the 1970 survey, only 16% were men. As mentioned, the agoraphobic phase of an anxiety state in a man may be expressed as reluctance to travel from his home town, or to sit through long business meetings where, like so many agoraphobics, he finds the confinement difficult to endure. He feels trapped.

COLLAPSE

A sudden unexpected feeling of collapse can be almost as frightening as palpitations, especially when the weakness is further increased by panic.

Sensitisation is not a necessary prerequisite for an attack of weakness. It is not unusual for a busy person who has eaten little breakfast or gone without lunch to have a mild hypoglycaemic attack. It is surprising how often a first attack of hypoglycaemia occurs while the victim waits in a queue on the way home from work. The extra energy needed to stand after a tiring day, possibly under the added strain of being impatient, while waiting for a bus or train, may trigger the attack.

The first hypoglycaemic episode can be frightening, especially if it begins with that strange feeling of dissolution, almost approaching death, which often preludes the attack. I have been surprised at how many agoraphobics will confide, 'I was standing at the bus-stop and suddenly a strange feeling came over me, as if I was going to die. I felt weak and giddy and my heart started racing; my knees buckled under me. I panicked and could only just crawl on to a bus. When I reached home I was exhausted and since then I have not dared to travel alone.'

GIDDINESS

Few patients are easily convinced that such a disturbing physical condition as giddiness can be caused by nerves. The thought of brain tumour haunts many and even if persuaded that nerves are the culprit they dread going out while the houses seem to topple, the pavement to heave. Tension may so affect the sight that objects seem blurred and distant view is covered with a shimmering haze. Such a person may wait for days in the house for the giddiness to pass before daring to venture out. I have known some women to wait indefinitely, because as soon as they think of leaving the house, the tension mounts and giddiness returns.

One woman was haunted by the fear of being held up in her car by the red light at an intersection. As soon as the green changed to amber she would think, 'I daren't stop now! This is where I always have a dizzy spell.' So she would rush through the crossing on the amber light and, of course, the extra tension accentuated any tendency to giddiness.

SORROW AND DEPRESSION

A person in deep sorrow may cling to the house refusing to socialise. Also, from the strain of constant anxious brooding on his sorrow and perhaps with the added stress of malnutrition (he may only pick at his food), a sufferer could become debilitated and consequently sensitised and finally subjected to all the reactions sensitisation can bring, including agoraphobia.

Reluctance to move from home, even from the bed, can be part of any depression. Indeed, sometimes people not depressed have to force themselves to go out and many experience departure-blues before leaving on a voyage. Depression aggravates this normal feeling of reluctance to move away from home and, after depression lifts, memory of this reluctance may linger so vividly that reluctance to leave home may remain as an established habit.

NO APPARENT CAUSE

As mentioned, only 5.6% of patients in the 1970 survey could give no cause for their agoraphobia. In my practice, when a patient could give no cause for his illness – often claiming that panic had come unbidden – further questioning sometimes revealed that when panic first appeared the patient had been going through a stressful period and was therefore possibly sensitised. The pre-existing strain had become so overshadowed by the agoraphobia that it had been forgotten. It is physiologically impossible for panic to come unbidden.

ESTABLISHMENT

Surely it is understandable that a woman having these experiences prefers to stay at home or, if she must go shopping, takes someone with her for support, even a child. If she takes a child it may not be long before she becomes afraid that the child will see her 'like this', so she postpones shopping until an adult can accompany her.

If she does pluck up courage and ventures out alone, if only to the end of the street, she usually meets many obstacles on the way. Sensitisation and memory make her so aware of her nervous feelings, it is as if she is wearing headphones tuned in to her slightest reaction. Naturally, her autonomic nerves respond to this anxious introspection by becoming unusually alert so that it takes only some mild added strain to produce panic and perhaps the other symptoms of stress she dreads so much. Invariably she reacts by either turning and hurrying home or by grimly forcing her way forward. If she goes forward fighting, mounting tension may so stiffen her muscles that she may finally stand 'paralysed' – in the words of one woman, 'rooted to the ground' – perhaps holding on to the nearest support. Compulsion to return home becomes so strong she feels pulled forcibly back with every step she tries to take forward. For her, walking down the street is almost like trying to walk through a concrete wall.

She particularly dreads a big emporium because the crowd, heat, noise and absence of a place to rest confuse and invite 'that weak feeling'. Hot weather aggravates symptoms, because vasodilation increases hyperkinetic action and more readily brings consciousness of her heart's beating, thumping, of increased sweating and a feeling that her face will burst. Indeed she is convinced her illness shows on her face and to avoid scrutiny may prefer to wear dark glasses, go out at night or in the rain, when fewer people are about.

If a woman fighting her way forward manages to reach the supermarket, how natural when standing in a queue at the check-out to think, 'Wouldn't it be awful if I had a turn now, hemmed in like this!' Even if she escapes before panic and confusion strike too overwhelmingly, she remembers the experience so vividly she usually tries to avoid shopping alone in a supermarket in future; indeed she may become so afraid of the panic and other nervous sensations that she may avoid shopping alone anywhere. Some become so afraid they avoid travelling from home even if accompanied. They become housebound, established in severe agoraphobia. A few become so incapacitated by fear of having a turn, they will not stir as far as the clothes line to hang out clothes. Others will not take a bath if alone in the house.

In my opinion, until the importance of the havoc sensitisation alone can bring is recognised as a likely cause of some anxiety states and consequently of so much agoraphobia, the present rate of cure of both will not improve as much as it otherwise would. I stress again that in the vast majority of my agoraphobic patients the cause was neither deep-seated nor difficult to find. *Their agoraphobia was the result of severe sensitisation suddenly, or gradually, acquired and kept alive by bewilderment and fear.*

I have been surprised at the intensity with which some of my colleagues have defended their belief that an anxiety state is due either to some deep-seated cause (perhaps subconscious) or to some character inadequacy and that the illness can be cured only if such causes are found and treated. As already pointed out, sensitisation can come to anyone at any time, and to be bewildered by its acute and baffling symptoms is surely not unnatural. It is difficult to understand why the many people who respond in this natural way should be automatically thought inadequate, or why finding some deep-seated cause thought essential. Sensitisation can be shocking and confidence quickly shaken. One does not have to be a dependent type (as I have heard agoraphobics described) to be so affected. Some nervously ill doctors, with their medical training, fail to understand sensitisation or know how to cope with its effects on themselves (and I have seen this), so why should a layman be expected, as a matter of course, to be wise enough to do so?

Fear is one of our strongest and most disagreeable emotions; is it so inconceivable that a sensitised person could be afraid of its exaggerated expression in himself? Why cannot fear when it flashes almost electrically for so little cause or for no apparent reason – as it can in a sensitised person – be a cause in itself for the development of an anxiety state? In my experience with hundreds (I could say thousands) of patients in an anxiety state, it so often is.

Far from being dependent types many nervously ill people show courage and independence fighting their fears, often with little help from their families, and unfortunately sometimes without adequate understanding from their therapists.

So much depends on a therapist's ability to explain the nuances of this strange illness; for example, to explain why, when the patient is feeling better, setbacks can come for no apparent reason and be so especially devastating as if no progress had been made; to explain why symptoms thought forgotten can return acutely after months, years, of absence; why all the symptoms can then so quickly appear; why such demoralising exhaustion can so rapidly follow the return of symptoms; why, despite the right attitude, sensitisation may sometimes linger for such an unconscionably long time; why, when the agoraphobic returns home after being successful, it may seem that no success has been achieved and going out the next day be as difficult as ever. The 'whys' seem countless.

Unless the therapist has special understanding a pessimistic attitude towards curing agoraphobia is to be expected. An agoraphobic woman wrote of herself and her fellow sufferers, 'If unmarried, we're patted on the back and told we'll be better when we are. If married, that another baby will fix us; if middle-aged, it's the change!'

Also, too many patients are accused of escaping from responsibility by retreating into illness, especially agoraphobia. I have rarely met the agoraphobic man or woman who has no wish to recover. He may have failed so often in the attempt that his will to get better seems dead. However, it usually smoulders on and if suitably encouraged will rise again for another valiant effort.

Of course, some people have special problems and the strain of trying to cope with these may have sensitised them and helped to originate and maintain their illness. Naturally such problems must be coped with before complete recovery is possible. However, there are many people with no special problem other than possible lessened ability to cope with responsibilities because of illness, and I wish to highlight the importance of sensitisation in causing and inaintaining an anxiety state and any accompanying agoraphobia in these people.

Some therapists would admit the possibility that some people have a subconscious cause for their agoraphobia and need psychoanalysis. I do not close my mind to this possibility, but it is interesting that over thirty years of practice and curing many hundreds of agoraphobic people, it was not necessary for me to use psychoanalysis on any patient.

Of course, there is more to nervous illness than physical symptoms. Continuous tension accompanied by recurring panic can bring disconcerting experiences: indecision, suggestibility, loss of confidence, feelings of unreality, obsession, feelings of personality disintegration, depression. I discuss these and their logical development from chronic anxiety in a later chapter.

Part 2: Treatment

CHAPTER FOUR

The Four Concepts

My treatment is based on, first, adequate explanation to the patient of sensitisation and nervous symptoms; secondly, on teaching the importance of the four concepts – FACING, ACCEPTING, FLOATING, LETTING TIME PASS – and finally, on full explanation of the obstacles met during all stages of recovery and warning of the probable occurrence of setbacks and their treatment. Working this way many patients need no, or little, drug therapy.

This treatment is directed toward achieving desensitisation, by which I mean a reduction of exaggerated nervous sensations and emotional responses to normal intensity. Recovery lies not in the abolition of nervous sensations and feelings (as so many patients believe) but – as just stated – in their reduction to normal intensity.

The four concepts in more detail are:
    face – do not run away;
    accept – do not fight;
    float – do not tense;
    let time pass – do not be impatient with time.

These directions may sound almost too simple to be taken seriously; however, it is enlightening to see how many people sink deeper into nervous illness by doing the opposite.

The nervously ill person usually notices each new

symptom in alarm, listens-in in apprehension and yet, at the same time, is afraid to examine it too closely for fear of making it worse. He may agitatedly seek occupation to try to force forgetfulness. *He is running away*, not facing.

So many try to cope with unwelcome feelings by tensing themselves against them, thinking, 'I mustn't let this get the better of me!' When talking to another, the nervous person may clench his hands tightly, anxiously watching the clock, wondering how much longer he can keep up the masquerade without 'cracking'. *This is fighting*, not accepting.

Floating resembles accepting. It means to go with the feelings, offering no tense resistance, as one would if floating on calm water, letting the body move with the gentle undulation of the waves. It means loosening towards nervous sensations; letting the body go slack before them *as willingly as possible*. Some will say, 'How can I float past a whipping flash of panic?' They can by taking the panic with as little resistance as possible; by waiting until the flash spends itself and then going on with the job on hand. It is the letting go and consequent release from some tension implied by the word 'floating' that matters. Floating is the opposite to fighting. I have occasionally cured a patient in an anxiety state by using the simple words, 'Float. Don't fight!'

Also, the nervously ill person keeps looking back and worrying because so much time has passed in illness and he is not cured, as if there were an evil spirit that could be exorcised if only he, or the doctor, knew how. *He is impatient with time*, not willing to let time pass.

Agitated avoidance, the tension of fighting, the impatience with time, all add up to increased stress, increased sensitisation, prolonged illness.

After I have spoken about agoraphobia on radio and

television, the studio switchboard is frequently jammed with incoming calls from people who have heard themselves and their fears described for the first time. Many have said that acknowledgment that the origin of their illness could be simple, together with the detailed description of how they felt, with the added recognition of their fear of the symptoms of fear, was the reassurance they had wanted for so long and had despaired of finding. So often, the complicated reasons given to some of those who had previously sought help had only discouraged and disheartened. For example, an agoraphobic woman had been told that her reluctance to face the world was based on her subconscious knowledge that, as a child, she had been raped by her father. She said that these symptoms had first appeared soon after her husband had taken a mistress. She was eventually cured by losing her fear of the symptoms of stress by facing and accepting and letting time pass.

Fear of the symptoms of stress found in so many patients in an anxiety state with their anxiety complicated by agoraphobia makes treatment by behaviourism less successful for agoraphobia than for specific monosymptomatic phobias. Dr Marks[1], writing about 20 patients with severe agoraphobia whom he had treated by desensitisation, said, 'Attacks of panic and anxiety were the reason for poor results. Patients, who had recently overcome their fears, at times reported that a single panic might undo the effects of weeks of treatment and if less severe attacks of anxiety were repeated, the fear might also be relearnt. It was often extremely difficult to treat such attacks. . . Desensitisation produces only limited changes in severe agoraphobia.'

It is now becoming generally recognised that practical support in the places most feared helps some patients, and in some hospitals (for example, Warneford Hospital,

University of Oxford; Maudsley Hospital, London) nurse-therapists are being trained to accompany agoraphobic patients on practice journeys. However, for the best results, it is essential that the therapist should understand (as mentioned earlier) the many baffling aspects of agoraphobia, such as the exact meaning of recovery, the part memory plays in delaying recovery, the difficulties a patient meets in coming through setbacks; should also appreciate the incapacitating nature of agoraphobic panic and recognise that *the patient must learn how to cope with panic and not try to recover by simply 'getting used to' one difficult situation after another*. This is where teaching the concepts face, accept, float, is, in my opinion, essential.

For example, at a seminar at a London Hospital, a young nurse-therapist showed a video tape of his treatment of a middle-aged agoraphobic woman. The therapist persuaded the woman, who had not travelled alone for years, to walk around the block by herself. On her return he enquired how she had managed. She said, 'I didn't panic at all!' He answered, 'Good! Now I want you to do it again!' Surprised, she asked, 'Why?' 'It'll do you good!' he said. She set off reluctantly and returned shaky, afraid. The therapist asked her to repeat the journey several times, each time answering her 'Why?' with the same, 'It'll do you good!'

To show necessary understanding this therapist should have explained how and why the second journey would differ from the first; explained that she had not felt panic the first time round because she had walked on a cloud of part dream, part exhilaration at achieving the hitherto apparently unachievable; explained that on the second journey the dream would fade, that she would probably be only too aware of where she was, and that the distance would then seem greater and so give more occasion and time for panic. Such explanation would have given her more understanding of her illness, more confidence in the therapist, and would have earned her more willing co-operation during the more difficult tasks ahead.

Special understanding would also include the therapist's teaching the patient how to cope with panic and any other nervous symptom, or experience, encountered on those journeys around the block, and not to depend for cure on 'getting used to' walking alone. 'Getting used to' leaves the patient too vulnerable during future stress to the return of symptoms, especially panic. In other words, for lasting recovery, the therapist should teach the patient how to cope with the actual symptoms (see Chapter 5), not merely with a specific situation conducive to their occurence.

In private practice I encourage each new patient (man or woman) by telephone until I have him moving successfully from home. In the beginning this may mean daily contact for a few weeks (usually two) and thereafter less frequently. Before the agoraphobic leaves the house, I ask him to repeat to me how I want him to think about his illness and what I want him to do while out. It is essential that he understands clearly how he should cope with himself before he starts off to practise doing it. I also ask him to telephone me on his return. Contacting me after his big effort gives the patient tremendous encouragement, especially if no one is home to greet him. It also gives me opportunity to discuss his journey with him and this is rewarding to us both if he thinks the journey has been a failure, because I can usually point out his mistakes and persuade him to go out again immediately and turn failure at least into some semblance of success.

This treatment may sound too demanding to some therapists; however, I have found the comparatively quick recovery of patients treated in this way more than compensates for the extra time given. While a therapist's telephoning from an Out Patients' Department is less convenient than from a private surgery, it is not impossible and, again, the comparative quickness of recovery saves crowding an Out Patients' session with chronic agoraphobics.

In treatment by remote direction I substituted quarterly journals of encouragement for the telephoning.

Although it is not within the scope of this book to discuss nervously ill people with personality difficulties, conflicts and other problems, *simply understanding nervous symptoms and experiences* (as discussed in the following chapters) *and knowing how to cope with them helps such a person find some peace and so enables him to give more attention to any particular problem retarding recovery.*

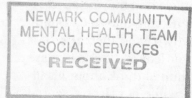

CHAPTER FIVE

Understanding and Coping with Symptoms

(1) Panic
(2) Palpitations
(3) Difficulty in expanding the chest
(4) Feeling of collapse
(5) Difficulty in swallowing
(6) Any new symptom

The person who has some problem helping to keep him sensitised must usually be released from this special stress before recovery can be complete. However, as mentioned earlier, this person usually finds some comfort, even some peace, from understanding and learning how to cope with his nervous symptoms.

For the person without a special problem, understanding the cause and nature of his symptoms is the beginning of cure. Too many nervously ill people say they have never had explanation of their symptoms and many of these recover when they get it. One man said, 'I did not believe it could be so simple. I feel I have been let out of prison.' This ignorance of patients previously treated (sometimes for years) before consulting me has given me the incentive to include the following simple explanations.

(1) PANIC

Cure of panic depends fundamentally on the patient's

understanding that sensitisation exaggerates the intensity of panic and that without the recurring lash of increasingly intense panic (reverberated circuits), nerves would calm and other nervous symptoms be less severe. The next step is to teach the patient how to desensitise himself.

As mentioned earlier, to avoid panicking while out the agoraphobic may arrange special props. Some women push a perambulator; other agoraphobics prefer to venture out at night, or in the rain, when they feel less conspicuous and expect to meet fewer people. Such subterfuge may support the sufferer enough to venture further and further from home, until he (or she) thinks himself cured. However, he does not fully understand how he has recovered and may have the constant, pressing thought, 'What if IT were to come back!' Since IT is fear, as long as he is afraid of its return, it has an open invitation to do so. Also props have a habit of giving way. *The surest way to permanent recovery is to know how to face and cope with panic and not placate it with subterfuge.*

The first step in treatment is to remove confusion by teaching the patient how to analyse and understand panic. He should know that when he panics he feels not one fear, as he supposes, *but two separate fears* – a first and second fear. The importance of recognising two separate fears cannot be over emphasised because, although the sensitised person may have no control over the first fear, with understanding and practice he can learn how to control the second fear and it is *this second fear that is keeping the first fear alive and so keeping the sufferer sensitised, ill.*

Most of us have experienced first-fear from time to time. It comes almost reflexly in response to danger, is normal in intensity and passes with the danger. However, the sensitised person's first-fear is so electric, so out of proportion to the danger causing it, he usually recoils from it, at the same time adding a second flash – *fear of the first-fear*.

Indeed, he may be much more concerned with the feeling of panic than with the original danger and because sensitisation prolongs first-fear, the second flash may seem to join it and so *the two fears feel like one*.

The flash of first-fear can come in response to anxiety only vaguely understood, to some mildly unpleasant memory or, as mentioned earlier, it may seem to come unbidden. Surely one can understand how easily victimised a sensitised person can be by first-fear.

All the symptoms that may come with fear, pounding heart, churning stomach and so on, can be called first-fear because these also seem to come unbidden and to them the nervously ill person adds plenty of second-fear. Recognising second-fear is made easier when the patient realises that it can be usually prefixed by 'What if?' or 'Oh, my goodness!' ('It took two capsules to get me to sleep last night, what if two don't work tonight?'). The agoraphobic woman hemmed in at the school meeting has only to feel trapped to flash first-fear and then to follow with second-fear as she thinks, 'Oh, my goodness, here it is again! I'll make a fool of myself in front of all these people! Let me out of here, quickly! Quickly!' With each 'quickly' tension and panic mount until she wonders how much longer she can hold on. So, she takes an even tighter, tenser, more sensitising grip on herself.

Mounting tension can be alarming and exhausting. It is difficult to hold tensely on to oneself for a short time and yet these people try to do so for an hour or more. Small wonder that as the panic grows they sense a crisis in which 'something terrible' will happen. As mentioned earlier, they are not quite sure what this something is, but they feel it hovering menacingly. They do not understand that it is the fears they add themselves – the succession of second-fears – that may finally drive them to find refuge outside the school hall.

Outside, they feel relieved, but when they realise that they have failed once more, they despair of ever being able to sit through another function. They gave themselves an impossible task; they went through every moment heroically *but they did it the wrong way.*

To cope and remain inside the hall, the agoraphobic must practise seeing panic through with as much acceptance as he can manage. He should be taught that panic can come only in a wave and must always die down *if he but waits* and does not fall into the trap of stoking his fires with second-fear. If he remains seated, takes a deep breath and lets it out slowly, lets his body loosen to the best of his ability (the deep breath and loosening encourage relaxation), even slumps in his chair and is prepared to let panic flash, *do its worst without withdrawing from it,* there will be no mounting panic. A sensitised body may continue to flash fear from time to time, but at least the sufferer will be able to see the function through. *The panic will not mount.* The realisation that they were being bluffed by no more than physical feelings of no great medical significance has cured some people.

If prepared to practise seeing panic through, such acceptance, shaky though it may be at first, brings enough peace to begin desensitisation. *It is the constant bombardment by second-fear for one reason or another that keeps nerves alerted, always triggered to fire (and fire is a good word) first-fear so intensely.*

Even when an agoraphobic succeeds in coping with second-fear, desensitisation takes time. With constant acceptance, a sensitised body usually continues to flash panic with exaggerated intensity for about two months.

However, few people can manage constant acceptance, so that each person must be prepared for his desensitisation to take its own special time.

Some complain that although they no longer panic they have a feeling of apprehension, almost of vibration, as if panic were 'just around the corner'. Patients understand this if it is compared to the vibrations of a bell after it has been struck and the sound has died away. When a patient understands, he is more able to accept the feeling and function with it there. A woman wrote, 'I soon learnt to disregard the inner trembling, vibration, that came instead of panic. It didn't last long!'

Sensitised nerves heal as naturally as a broken leg and just as naturally take time. It may seem an impossible demand for the sufferer to let time pass. Even with determination to accept, he may think himself too exhausted to do so. It is as if his mind were willing but his body too tired to obey the mind's commands. For such a person (too often the exhausted housewife) two or three weeks with extra tranquillisation may be necessary. There is still stigma attached to having been in a psychiatric hospital which some people find hard to live down. So, if possible, I arrange sedation in a patient's home or in the home of one of his relatives. I especially avoid hospitalisation for a patient who has previously experienced it.

Recently a mother of a patient telephoned to say her daughter was in a 'shocking state' of confusion. She said, 'The last time she was like this the doctor put her into hospital immediately. Must this happen again?' The young woman was 28 and had been in and out of hospital from the age of 17. I first saw her two years ago and since then she had progressed enough to undertake a course of study. Unfortunately the course was too strenuous (four subjects, each at a high level) for one who had not studied for so long. She became overanxious, overworked and finally mentally fatigued.

Although confused, she understood enough to be upset by failure and to dread returning to hospital. However, sedation and almost continuous sleep at home for two days cleared the confusion. She gained confidence when she saw that confusion can be caused by fatigue, that she was not going 'mental' and that she could recover without being sent back to hospital. In my opinion, to have read-mitted her to hospital would have been a mistake.

A patient may be so far improved he may experience quite severe flashes of panic and other nervous symptoms and yet, at the same time, feel they no longer matter. One woman said, 'I still suffer from agoraphobic symptoms but I'm not afraid of them any more. They are just a nui-sance.' The feelings linger because of memory and habit working together on some remaining sensitisation. *Recovery lies not so much in the absence of symptoms, as in knowing how to cope with those present.* That woman was closer to recovery than one whose symptoms had left her without her understanding how or why.

The patient should be taught the difference between ac-ceptance and just 'putting up with'. 'Putting up with' means hoping panic will come quickly and 'get it over'; it means limiting moving to places where the sufferer thinks he will not panic, so that his horizon becomes narrower and narrower until it is eventually bounded by the front door. 'Putting up with' means continued illness.

True acceptance means recognising second-fear and adding as little as possible. When the patient is familiar with second-fear he will be amazed at how much he has been adding as torture to his daily life. *True acceptance means even welcoming panic as an opportunity to practise coping with it as taught until it no longer frightens.*

I have watched many patients come through panic to peace and find lasting cure, even those who thought they were cowards. A small committee was responsible for the financial management and distribution of the quarterly journals mentioned in Chapter 1. The Honorary Assistant Secretary wrote, 'A year ago I would not have thought that I would be writing a progress report. At that time I was so deeply involved in a major setback that to walk a few paces from my front door was enough to bring all the old terrifying symptoms, and so failure piled upon failure.

'However, with the support of the journals I managed somehow to carry on practising in a very feeble way. I was frequently in such deep despair, I felt that even the little effort I was making was too much for my strength, especially as I seemed to get nowhere. The prospect of giving up altogether was tempting, although this too filled me with a feeling of hopelessness.

'This is where it becomes important to remember to let time pass. After some months, I began to win small victories and was able to look back from one week to another and see that I had progressed, although there were still dark days; but after more time, these became fewer. One day I was actually able to say I felt better, more at ease. At this stage, progress seemed to speed up (the word 'speed' is purely relative here!) although it was some time before bad days did not happen any more.

'Now I feel relaxed and free to move around. I will not pretend that I haven't still a long way to go, but I can view the prospect with optimism. How glad I am I didn't give up. To fellow sufferers I would say, "Never give up. Keep practising and letting time pass." Some of you will think, "Oh, yes. It's alright for her to talk but I couldn't do it!" but I know you can, because I have come up from just those depths of suffering that you are in now and *courage was never one of my strong points!'*

Sensitised panic rarely vanishes by simply ceasing to come. It goes only when the panic is taken out of panic; that is, by the patient's seeing panic through the right way so often, without adding second-fear, that eventually panic loses so much of its fire that the remainder no longer matters. To try to switch panic off, avoid its coming, alleviate it with drugs, brings no permanent cure. The patient is too vulnerable to returns of panic which can shock him into utter despair. This is why treatment by simultaneous sedation and suggestion to rid a patient of fear in some dreaded situation (a form of behaviourism), while useful for single phobias, may fail for agoraphobia. As mentioned earlier, the person with a monosymptomatic fear is afraid of a specific object outside himself. The agoraphobic is afraid of the upsetting physical feelings he feels within himself when in certain situations. He must be taught to cope with these feelings, not with a situation, otherwise he may manage one dreaded situation after another only to panic in a new one.

Recently I saw a video-taped session of an agoraphobic man being taken by a nurse-therapist on journeys in a local bus. The patient had already had a series of treatments in fantasy with little result. The programme was now for active treatment. The patient asked only to be able to travel in a bus to his work.

After repeated journeys with the therapist, the man achieved his wish. When I asked the therapist on what principle he had helped the patient, he answered, 'No particular principle; I suppose he just got used to going on a bus!' Now, if the time ever came when that man should be temporarily obliged to stop his daily rides (for example, through illness), travelling alone again could be as difficult as ever. With no guide-line to help him except 'getting used to', he could panic severely and undo months of previous effort. *It is essential that the patient be taught how to cope with panic.*

The Ultimate

Much suffering is caused by ignorance and in particular by the hovering shadow of having to one day face what some sufferers call 'the ultimate'. Few can describe exactly what they mean by this, but each is convinced it is crucial.

The following excerpt is from a tape recording I made for a woman agoraphobic for 28 years (Chapter 8), who repeatedly mentioned fear of facing the ultimate (her word):

DOCTOR: 'You are still making the mistake of being put off by what you imagine might happen. You should try to concentrate on what is actually happening. At your present stage of illness, a certain amount of flashing panic seems to come automatically, but some comes because you have not yet had the courage often enough to face and pass through what you call the ultimate.

'Your idea of the ultimate is a crisis that lies beyond the peak of panic. You can't picture this clearly, but it threatens like some final explosion of agitation and fear. Your imagined ultimate is only a state of supertension of your own making. When you pluck up the courage to go toward it *willingly*, it melts because even the small amount of relaxation in the slightest willingness is enough to release some tension. You then pass through the supertension you have been building up for yourself. In other words you disperse the ultimate.

'Practise, practise, practise. Take your journey moment by moment. Regard it as moments to be passed through, not a threatening distance to be covered. Don't think, "I *will* get there!" and then struggle to do it without panicking. PANIC, but practise passing through panic without adding second-fear. It is the panic, the moment of crisis – the ultimate if you like to call it that – that you must learn to cope with, *not the distance*.

'See each crisis through slowly; no rush. So now drive on [this woman was practising driving alone] quietly, moment by moment. Go forward with the car. When you panic try to put into words what you feel – don't withdraw dumbly, blindly, from an imagined terror, an imagined ultimate! And never turn back. You are so far advanced toward recovery, you have learnt that if you turn back you are disappointed and obliged to return and repeat the journey. Why waste time? So, go on gently, slowly, willingly, ready to accept all, especially that threatening crisis you call the ultimate.'

A patient may say, 'I have been given two different kinds of advice. First, to let fear come and do its worst and face it until it no longer matters and, second, to relax and so reduce the stress which will then reduce the panic. Which advice am I to follow?' These two statements are fundamentally the same. When the sufferer is prepared to face panic and accept, he automatically lets go in attitude and this brings enough relaxation to eventually lessen emotional reaction. Resignation brings a certain peace. The clue to failure or success lies in attitude.

(2) PALPITATIONS AND 'MISSED' HEARTBEATS
A surprising number of people say they were precipitated into an anxiety state and then into agoraphobia by some sudden unexpected, and hitherto unexperienced, frightening and yet usually harmless, physical sensation such as

a first attack of palpitations. It is not enough to be told, 'It's only nerves.' More reassurance comes from the doctor's stressing the size and strength of the heart muscle and the impossibility of its 'bursting'; from explaining that nervous palpitations are only a temporary upset in the timing of the heartbeats; that 'missed' beats are not truly missed, are merely beats spaced irregularly with the timing again at fault and that the heart compensates for an unusually quick beat by taking a restful pause, so that the beat following the long pause if therefore naturally forceful, so the heart seems to thump. To a sensitised person each extrasystole can feel as disconcerting as the jerk of a sudden descent in a lift – uncomfortable indeed when he is subjected to long runs of extrasystoles.

To know that the thumping, racing, nervous heart is still under control, that it will not stop beating and will always revert to normal rhythm, helps the patient regain confidence and take his heart's unusual beating more philosophically. Patients deserve explicit explanations.

(3)   DIFFICULTY IN EXPANDING THE CHEST
The patient may say he cannot expand his chest enough to take in a deep breath. In the words of one woman, 'I pant and gasp for air.' This is another reason why so many avoid sitting in a crowded hall (not enough oxygen there!). I explain that nature was not so foolish as to put into our conscious control the full responsibility of breathing, otherwise how would we breathe when asleep, or under an anaesthetic? I describe how the respiratory centre automatically regulates breathing according to the concentration of carbon dioxide in the blood. To illustrate this, I ask the patient to see how long he can hold his breath. At first he may be reluctant to try 'such a

dangerous experiment', but when he does he is surprised to find that after about half a minute he is forced, almost against his will, to take a very deep breath indeed.

When he appreciates the control beyond his control, he often sees the folly of his struggle, especially when I explain that his apparent inability to expand his chest is no more than tension of chest muscles.

I also point out how shallow breathing can wash out too much carbon dioxide, cause giddiness, make hands tingle and even go into a tetanic spasm. I also explain how the respiratory centre adjusts the level of carbon dioxide by slowing down breathing.

I hesitate to describe such an elementary procedure; however I am reminded of a young woman, suffering from hyperventilation, sent to me by her general practitioner. She walked into my surgery in obvious distress and said she had been breathing this way on and off for a year. She explained that although the cause of the original attack had passed, the habit of breathing this way had remained. After explanation and the breath-holding experiment described above, she left, breathing normally. Months later her practitioner reported that she was cured. He had tried every remedy he knew except simple explanation and demonstration.

(4) FEELING OF COLLAPSE

A patient understands nervous weakness more easily when it is compared to the weakness he would feel if suddenly told he had inherited a fortune. Understanding is further helped by explaining how, in shock, bloodvessels may dilate so that blood drains into dependent parts of the body, thus depriving the brain of blood and causing faintness.

The agoraphobic woman may have spasms of panic

(slight shock) whenever she thinks of going out alone, so that when she starts off she already feels weak and the extra strain of crossing a main road, boarding a bus, standing in a queue, may bring on those 'jelly legs'. She may think, 'What's the use of trying to go out today!' and return home. Surely it is not difficult to understand why, if she eventually ventures out again, she begins by timidly testing herself to see if she can get as far as the gate, then into the street and so on.

Of course, the fear she feels while testing is an invitation to the weakness she dreads. She has placed herself in a fear–adrenalin–fear cycle. To such patients I use the phrase, 'Jelly legs will get you there, if you will let them,' and explain that when legs feel this way, they are responding normally to a build-up of tension from her own fear and that the weakness and leaden feeling are not symptoms of true organic illness, are only feelings, and that she should try not to be bluffed by feelings however upsetting they may seem.

The patient keeps the best grip on himself by releasing it and abandoning himself to whatever nervous reaction his body may bring. This is difficult for him to believe, but it should be explained that by doing this he releases some of the tension that fatigues nerves controlling blood-vessels, muscles and nervously induced weakness comes less readily.

While the patient listens to his therapist he may be hopeful and ready to face the worst. However, it is not easy to stay reassured by his own reassurance during an attack of weakness away from home, especially if he has increased it by first panicking. Also, because of previous months, years of illness, weak spells may return from time to time despite understanding and acceptance.

I have already discussed (Chapter 3) the importance

of hypoglycaemia in causing a feeling of collapse. Its explanation and treatment are simple and well known by therapists.

Vasovagal attacks are rare in nervous illness; however, a therapist should have them in mind because they can come without preliminary symptoms and alarm the sufferer exceedingly, especially if he collapses in a dangerous place – such as while crossing a main road. I have seen blood pressure fall so low in a vasovagal attack that the patient was cyanosed, genuinely unable to move, almost unable to breathe. The attack should be treated energetically and the therapist should always be on the alert to differentiate between it and simple nervous weakness.

(5) DIFFICULTY IN SWALLOWING

A feeling of having a lump in the throat may be so troublesome that the sufferer may be sure he cannot swallow solid food, or at least find swallowing difficult. I keep biscuits in my surgery. When I ask such a patient to chew one he usually recoils and says he couldn't possibly swallow a biscuit. I point out that I said 'chew', not 'swallow', and while he reluctantly chews I warn against his swallowing. However, as soon as the moistened, softened biscuit reaches the back of his tongue, his swallowing reflexes take over and at least some of the biscuit is on its way down. I have cured anorexia nervosa in this way. A young girl with anorexia nervosa was almost hysterical because she was sure she would never be able to swallow again. In her words, 'At a point in my illness, I was convinced I would die. I could not swallow. However, my doctor took some strawberries and said, "Chew! Just chew! Don't try to swallow." I chewed. I had to accept the feeling of sickness, accept the fear and chew. To my surprise, the strawberries slipped down. I had not been conscious of swallowing. I followed this advice many times until gradually my stomach no longer rejected food.'

Her anorexia had started during a stressful time at home. Relief from this stress helped her recovery; however, for complete recovery she needed to overcome the physical difficulty of swallowing.

(6)   ANY NEW DISTURBING SYMPTOM

A patient should be warned against being impressed by any new disturbing symptom. From time to time he will probably visit his doctor with some normal physiological sensation that has been exaggerated by sensitisation until it has become uncomfortable, disconcerting. After reassurance that the trouble is nervous and (we hope) suitable explanation of its cause, he should try to accept it and understand that he will be easily impressed by a new symptom because he has been frightened for so long that being afraid is now a habit; fear like his will come at the slightest encouragement and cannot be banished overnight. For some time he may add second-fear almost reflexly, especially at the appearance of a new symptom. In the early stages of recovery he can only practise not adding second-fear and, when he fails, he must learn not to despair too much, not to expect too much from himself at this stage. The person who eventually recovers has learnt to disregard failure, despair.

The symptoms I have described are among those most often complained of by agoraphobic people. Other symptoms – churning stomach, blurred vision, trembling and so on – may occur and also have a simple explanation when nervous in origin. I stress again the urgent necessity to explain nervous symptoms.

CHAPTER SIX

Unravelling the Maze of Nervous Experiences

(1) Indecision
(2) Suggestibility
(3) Loss of confidence
(4) Feelings of unreality
(5) Obsession
(6) Feelings of personality disintegration
(7) Depression

Apart from the physical symptoms, the nervously ill person, whether agoraphobic or not, may have some strange experiences: indecision, suggestibility, loss of confidence, feelings of unreality, obsession, feelings of personality disintegration, depression.

These may appear much in the order stated, one leading to the other and, in so many of my patients, each based on sensitisation exaggerating emotional reaction and for some of the experiences – for example, obsession – the addition of mental fatigue.

The explanation that these experiences are based on sensitisation exaggerating emotional reaction, with the possible addition of mental fatigue, may seem too simple. However, I do not hesitate to affirm that they developed in this way in many of my patients without the complication of any deep-seated cause or any known specific problem originating and prolonging their illness. *The therapist should always be alerted to the physical effects of sensitisation* and know that, in the severely sensitised person, *all emotions can be exaggerated* – in a happy moment he may feel almost hysterical, and a mildly unhappy event may seem tragic. For example, a medical student in an acute anxiety state said that to see an old woman in the Out Patients' Department with no more than chronic bronchitis upset him so much he thought perhaps he should give up studying medicine.

I do not mean that the sensitised person's only problem is his sensitised state. Any problem that arises during his illness can, because of his vulnerability to exaggerated emotional reaction, assume exaggerated importance; for example, coping with the old woman with chronic bronchitis. Also, any problem or conflict he has kept suppressed enough to live with successfully while well may now raise its head and seem devastating, unmanageable and certainly adds to, and prolongs, his illness. Indeed, he may cope with one intruder only to be confronted with another.

The point I wish to make is that it is not solely the nature of the problem – if the patient has one – that is important in causing nervous experiences (indecision, suggestibility and so on). A therapist must be aware of, and treat, the exaggerated emotional response to it, as well as try to solve the problem.

(1) INDECISION

The slightest change of mind while trying to decide may be accompanied by such intense emotional reaction in the nervously ill that deciding may seem impossible. Each different point of view seems right one moment and equally wrong the next. Even trying to decide to take an umbrella may cause agitation. The umbrella will be down the path one minute and back in the hall the next.

It is not enough to tell such a person that, with practice, deciding will become easier. If he does occasionally make a decision without too much effort, while he remains sensitised, his emotions will continue to swing too readily with each changing point of view and decisions continue to be difficult.

(2) SUGGESTIBILITY

Because a nervously ill person has difficulty in making up his own mind, he becomes abnormally susceptible to the suggestions of others. He thinks that any suggestion that brings such strong emotional reaction as he feels must be important, even true. Reading a newspaper or magazine is a hazard. Pessimistic articles on recovery from nervous illness can affect the reader enough to send him into setback, especially the thoughtless pseudo-medical article about agoraphobia being incurable.

A young girl asked, 'Why do the wrong ideas come with such force and the right ones seem so shaky?' The wrong ideas come with force because they so often carry threat and so produce fear, one of our strongest emotions. The right ideas seem shaky because in a nervously ill person the forceful wrong ideas displace them so quickly and easily that they come only in glimpses. This is why hope, so desperately needed, is usually tentative.

Because the nervously ill person is so suggestible, his own suspicion that he may never recover can be devastating.

(3)   LOSS OF CONFIDENCE

Indecision and suggestibility must inevitably lead to loss of confidence. This logical development can be appreciated when one understands how exaggerated flashing emotion can confuse and delude.

A nervously ill person does not necessarily lack confidence at all times, he may swing suddenly to elated confidence and just as suddenly to despair. This in itself confuses. There is no middle of the road for him. As one woman expressed it, 'Sometimes I feel I'd rather stay down all the time, than swing up one minute and down the next!'

A man describing his loss of confidence said, 'The last day before returning home from holiday, there I was contemplating, "Will I go fishing or not?" I thought, "It's too rough!" It wasn't rough. I was trying to delude myself. All of a sudden I thought, "I'm going!" I went on my own and had a most exhilarating time. I caught a lot of fish and coming home I deliberately let the boat roll about in the sea and I can remember wading, pushing it ashore in front of me with fantastic energy, when only two hours earlier, I'd been shaking like a jelly at the thought of going.' He added quietly, 'Over this you really have to distrust your own judgement, haven't you?'

I explained that he had good reason to mistrust the advice he had been giving himself during those years of illness. Those were the obstructive messages that had kept him ill, and this was why I taught floating past such obstructive thought.

That man was second-in-charge of an important State industry. He had refused promotion to managing director because of agoraphobia of 40 years' standing. Many of my patients held responsible positions before they became ill, and had shown great courage struggling for years to keep working while feeling as inadequate as their illness made them feel. To regain confidence, these people needed mainly understanding of sensitisation and a programme for desensitisation. Return of confidence usually follows as acceptance and time desensitise and emotional reaction becomes normal. Of course, if nervous illness has been caused by the stress of worrying about personal failure, confidence lost in this way must be regained by more directed effort.

Often the person recovered from nervous illness reads, or hears, that because he has had a breakdown he is vulnerable to future breakdown. However, if he has recovered through his own effort based on understanding, he can not only rise above this upsetting suggestion, but can even appreciate that he could be less vulnerable to breakdown in the future than many people who have not had his illuminating experience.

Recently during an interview on radio, together with another physician and a psychiatrist, I mentioned, several times, patients recovering from nervous illness. The psychiatrist interrupted, saying, 'You speak of recovery from nervous illness. Surely you mean remission? One does not use the word recovery in connection with nervous illness!' Over the last 40 years I have seen so many recover from nervous illness (anxiety state) that I am not afraid to speak of recovery.

(4) FEELINGS OF UNREALITY

Depersonalisation and derealisation occur in 37% of the agoraphobics in the series of Harper and Roth[8]. Dr Marks[1] quotes their report: 'The patient feels temporarily strange, disembodied, cut off or far away from her immediate surroundings or feels that some change has occurred in her environment. The change referred to herself is called depersonalisation, while the same change referred to her surroundings is called derealisation. Depersonalisation and derealisation are equivalent . . . depersonalisation is a temporary, phasic, phenomenon, lasts a few seconds or minutes, or several hours. Its onset and termination are generally abrupt . . . the onset can follow some situation of extreme anxiety.'

I use the term unreality to include depersonalisation and derealisation because my patients understand and use it when describing similar experiences. Some say the feeling comes in flashes, others that there may be days when they feel fairly constantly withdrawn, unreal.

Feeling unreal is understandable when one considers how introspective a nervously disturbed person may become, paying less and less attention to the outside world, even to his immediate surroundings. We all know, when desperately concerned with our own affairs, how difficult it can be to pay due attention to outside events. It is even more difficult for the nervously ill to detach himself from his almost obsessive self-examination. The outside world naturally seems to recede as his interest in it decreases. In the words of one man, 'It is as if a grey veil separates me from people, things!'

This man described his first feeling of unreality. On one occasion when going for a swim, he had to pass from the bathing shed through a dark tunnel before emerging on to the beach. The sudden contrast between the darkness of the tunnel and the brilliance of the sunshine on the white sand and coloured umbrellas was so arresting that he suddenly felt forcibly drawn out of himself and said that only then did he realise how bound within his own thoughts he had been during the last weeks. The crowd of laughing people seemed in a world apart, as if on a stage (derealisation). The more he tried to be part of the scene, the further it receded. He became alarmed at the thought of the mental state he must be in and fled in fear. From then on a feeling of unreality was one of his main complaints. Had he understood the strangeness as the natural result of so much anxious brooding and had he not tried to lose it by fleeing from it, it would have gradually passed. A feeling of unreality, born as it is from tension and excessive introspection, will die from lack of attention.

However, it may take months for a nervously ill person to be refreshed enough by peace to be interested in everyday life. Much nervous suffering develops from continuous anxious introspection which entrenches disturbing thoughts in a mind made 'non-resilient' by fatigue.

The nervously ill person can feel unreal in different ways. Some say, 'I feel outside myself looking down at myself,' or, 'When I touch things I know I'm doing it but I can't *feel* I am!' Again, 'It doesn't seem real to hear people laughing,' or, 'I listen to people talking and half the time I see their mouths move and can't understand what they're saying. It's like looking at T.V. with the sound turned off.'

A mother was explaining on the telephone how difficult it was to understand the unreality she felt toward her young daughter. She said that even when she kissed the child goodnight, she felt she was kissing her in a dream. While she was talking, I heard a commotion in the background. Suddenly the mother shouted, 'Be quiet, Jean!' I pointed out that she had just experienced a very real moment of exasperation. She saw the point, and also understood when I explained that she had many such moments with her daughter but was so used to them that they hardly registered. The frightening moments of unreality blotted out the real moments. In her sensitised state, her fear of the feeling of unreality was so great that it soon replaced any peace my explanation brought. Tape recordings were essential to keep her reassured.

The illusion of loss of contact with the world can be further encouraged for some people by their losing any feeling of love for those they know they should love. They have felt intense fearful emotion for so long that normal emotions seem frozen. It is useless to try to force awareness of feeling and a waste of time analysing the patient to try to find a deep-seated cause of this condition. It is a symptom of emotional depletion.

When the patient understands the cause of unreality as the result of too much anxious introspection, he may be so relieved that he is not going mad that he may lose his feeling of unreality, and feel exhilaratingly real – too exhilaratingly, because this new feeling is usually short-lived. It is natural that unreality should return; memory alone will bring it. Unfortunately the sufferer may then be too easily led into thinking that the cause, in him, must be deep-seated indeed.

If a feeling of unreality is part of suffering, the sufferer should be taught to accept it as a natural consequence of his illness and to understand that, as he becomes less bewildered and introspection eases, he will become automatically more interested in outside events and will feel more closely related to them.

Recession

One woman described how, in moments of severe panic, she seemed to recede into her own mind toward 'a black nothingness'. This sensation was sometimes accompanied by a gripping pain in the head and ringing in the ears. She was sure that if this feeling were to continue further she would 'never come back' (become insane). Other patients complained of a similar experience in moments of intense panic. Recession is merely supertension added to superpanic.

The nervously ill person is easily influenced by his feelings of the moment. They are hard to bear and make such a deep impression that they assume inflated importance.

(5) OBSESSION

A fatigued mind may race agitatedly or work so slowly the sufferer may grope for thoughts. The tired mind may also seem to lose resilience so that frightening thoughts may seem to cling tenaciously. The bewildered sufferer often makes the mistake of trying to push away unwelcome thoughts or replace them with other thoughts. The more he fights in this way, the tenser he becomes and the more stubbornly thoughts seem to cling. Discarding unwelcome thoughts can be difficult at any time for anyone. For example many of us know the difficulty of getting a tune off our mind when overtired. And yet, the obsessive person constantly demands this of himself. Small wonder he despairs as he tries to find ways to keep unwanted thoughts at bay. Many obsessions begin this way: *an unwanted habit established by exaggerated emotional reaction to some frightening thought in a mentally fatigued person.*

A woman described the effects of fatigue on her obsessions during an experience she had before becoming my patient. She said, 'In addition to my other obsessions, I developed a fear of harming others and going mad. I daren't tell anyone. I couldn't sleep. I became sick at the drop of a hat and when in the depths of horror, although I felt frozen, I was sweating and not so much trembling as shuddering violently. I know now that this was shock and that it was brought on by utter fatigue and fear. When I told them at the hospital that I was shocked, they didn't understand and kept asking, "Aren't you depressed?" My doctor advised shock treatment. He said it worked for depression; but I wasn't depressed. However, I agreed to have the treatment and it helped me, but I suspect not in quite the way they thought. The doctor gave me an injection to put me to sleep before treatment and for 20 minutes, I had peace – just nothing, for 20 minutes. When I came round, all I could say, over and over, was "I've been asleep!" I felt so grateful. *I'm sure that obsessive illness is somewhere tied up with mental tiredness.'*

To some patients the nature of obsession is secondary to the horror of the habit of 'being like this'; for example, repeating a tune or number is not frightening in itself, but being obliged to do it is very frightening. To others the type of obsession is important. For example, the nervously ill mother is naturally afraid of accidentally harming her child, while, because of illness, she lacks confidence and concentration. She may remember having read about a woman harming her baby on purpose and she may be so horrified at her own fear of harming her child that the thought that she may do so accidentally may become the fear that she will do so purposely. Overwhelming horror in a fatigued, suggestible mind is fertile soil for the development of obsessions.

Such a woman is not necessarily an aggressive type, as so many of my patients suffering this way had been previously told by a former therapist. She is no more than a frightened mother with an illness that brings this not uncommon obsession. So many mothers have this fear of harming their child, surely they cannot all be aggressive. To brand a nervously ill woman aggressive not only does not help, but upsets her unnecessarily and makes recovery more difficult. Unfortunately such a woman is too easily convinced that she must be peculiar, because in her depleted state she may have reached the stage where she no longer feels love for the child. It is paradoxical that, as mentioned earlier, although nervously ill people may feel frightening emotions intensely, other emotions may seem deadened.

While some nervously ill people find help in religion, to

others it brings no comfort. This can cause havoc in a person dedicated to a religious life, especially when he is plagued by what he thinks are sinful thoughts. Thoughts can be grotesque in an abnormally anxious person when accompanied by mental fatigue. The more strange, unreal, sinful, they seem, the more the sufferer may feel compelled to pursue them as if mesmerised to find out just how horrible they can be. However grotesque, these thoughts are to be expected in the sufferer's present state and he should not feel guilty, or fear them as something to be avoided, as if there were parts of his brain he dare not use. Above all, he should not give them undue importance by taking them seriously. *It does not matter how much the sufferer dwells on his obsessions if he does so willingly.* He must be taught how to see all thoughts for what they are, *only thoughts*, and shrink from none of them, however severe the compulsion that accompanies them. Severe tension can give such force to some thoughts that they seem to lock their victim in submission. Release from even a little tension by release from some of the fear through acceptance helps to 'unlock' the 'locked' mind.

The common habit of trying to replace unwelcome thought with other thoughts is more likely to entrench an obsession than cure it. Yet the advice to substitute in this way is sometimes given. For example, the following extract was published recently by a well-established Australian self-help organisation in one of its handbooks under the heading '*How to Control Undesirable Thoughts*': 'Crowd them out by cultivating positive thoughts, wholesome interests and habits.' This may sound good advice; however, trying to crowd out undesirable thoughts with positive thoughts can agitate. It also carries the fighting attitude, to which I am so opposed. The same pamphlet advised, 'Disregard by not voicing or acting on them [the thoughts].' Here again, if a person with obsessions had 'not acting on them' under his control he may not be considered obsessive. If the obsessive handwasher did not have to act according to his thoughts, there would be little left to cure. Cultivating positive thought and action to crowd out obtrusive thought gives far too much prominence to disturbing thoughts and so complicates illness. Effort to disregard is another way of regarding.

While the obsessive patient may understand what is expected of him, he usually finds accepting willingly very difficult. To give more help I teach him to *glimpse*. For example, if the obsession is constant handwashing for fear of contamination by germs, I explain how skin has natural oil to protect it and that constant washing removes this and makes the skin more vulnerable to infection. I then encourage the patient to try to glimpse and hold this point of view. In the beginning, his obsession may be so severe he may be unable even to glimpse this truth. A few sessions practising glimpsing are not enough. Repetition of practice is the crux of treatment. So, again I make tape recordings. When the patient can finally glimpse the right point of view, repetition eventually strengthens belief in this point of view until it replaces the obsessive message.

At the first attempts at practising glimpsing, the obsessive thought may intrude so forcibly that thinking clearly, even for a flashing moment, is difficult, may seem impossible. The sufferer may be able to glimpse only when calmed by listening to his therapist or to a recording of his therapist's instructions. When he can glimpse by himself recovery has begun. Even so, he may be able to glimpse one minute and not the next. There will be hours, even days, when his ability to glimpse seems lost and having once experienced the hope that glimpsing brings, losing it can make the obsession seem worse.

Glimpsing can also help a patient with a problem. He should discuss the problem with a counsellor, find an acceptable way of looking at it and practise glimpsing it from this new point of view. A problem constantly viewed in an upsetting way becomes so 'engraven' on the mind that the sufferer has difficulty seeing it from any other point of view, so that it finally seems insoluble.

I have known a patient get temporary relief from an obsession by asking a companion to put into words the truth as he should be seeing it; the sufferer may even instruct his companion on the exact words to use. Hearing words spoken, even in this prearranged way, can release enough tension to enable the patient to glimpse truth and hold it, if only for a few moments. If capable of being helped like this, the patient usually already understands glimpsing, and realises that more time must pass before his fatigue lifts sufficiently, his emotional reactions calm and his mind becomes 'flexible' enough for him to reason successfully with himself.

The first experience of glimpsing successfully may come like a revelation. The woman who described earlier how she stood shocked before her obsessions later wrote, 'When I had my first glimpse, I could see my obsession for what it was – a silly thought in a tired mind – and if one thought could be silly, they all could be. It seemed as if the gates of heaven had opened. At this moment, nine months after my first glimpse, I can glimpse well. I started to make progress from the moment I understood glimpsing. I went down in patches, but nothing serious. In June or July, I had my first major setback. Looking back now it started with tiredness, not being able to sleep, worry over family illness and so on. I lost the ability to glimpse, but I stuck to my guns, took it as willingly as I could and went through. I'm better. Pennies are dropping everywhere now.' That woman had been plagued by obsessions for 17 years.

One may criticise glimpsing as treating the symptom, not the disease. In my experience, as far as the anxiety state is concerned, the disease is so often caused by fear of the symptoms. Sensitisation fosters development of obsessions and to try to cure them by analysing the patient to find an original cause for an obsession, while failing to recognise the presence and importance of accompanying sensitisation, is more often bound to fail than to succeed. Also, in a state of fear and mental fatigue, one obsession lost can be quickly replaced by another. The patient does not go looking for a new obsession; he is in a mentally fatigued state when any frightening thought can become fixed in his mind.

It is more the fear that accompanies the obsession that exhausts and resensitises than obeying, or trying not to obey, it; for example, persistent handwashing, although tiring in itself, is exhausting only when accompanied by fear of the habit. When the sufferer understands obsession as a combination of fatigue and exaggerated emotional response to fear, obsession may lose some of its nightmarish quality.

Unfortunately, few recognise the insidious approach of mental fatigue or know the tricks it can play. A student more readily understands; he knows that, after three or four hours of study, concentrating and remembering clearly become increasingly difficult and that he must stop working until mentally refreshed. The nervously ill person studies himself with little rest; he is so insistently drawn to self-study, he does not recognise the gradual onset of fatigue.

To an agoraphobic, fear of leaving the safety of home is often the most upsetting part of his anxiety state and, by staying at home as much as possible, he may live for weeks without excessive stress. This could explain why obsessions, although sometimes present, are not common among agoraphobics.

(6) FEELINGS OF PERSONALITY DISINTEGRATION

Surely it is not surprising for a nervously ill person to say that he feels as if his personality is disintegrating, or has disintegrated, when he finds it difficult to make a decision, easily falls victim to suggestion, has no confidence, is bewildered by unreality and perhaps by obsession and is buffeted by exaggerated physical symptoms of stress. He feels he has no inner strength on which to depend; no inner self from which to seek direction; no inner harmony holding thought and action together.

Old sayings are surprisingly apt when applied to nervous illness. 'Pull yourself together' describes so well what such a person thinks he should do, but cannot. It is as if he must gather the scattered pieces of his personality together and fit them into place, just as one would fit the scattered pieces of a jigsaw puzzle, before he can be himself again.

A young, nervously ill, resident doctor came for help. He was in such a state of emotional turmoil from fear, tension and bewilderment at the state he was in, that to steady himself enough to give a simple injection at the hospital had become a battle. Each day was spent fighting such battles. He felt exhausted. He used the term disintegrated when describing how he felt.

I explained the reason for his apparent disintegration – exaggerated emotional reaction through sensitisation accompanied by the agitation of excessive tension – and emphasised that he could continue at work only if, instead of meeting each situation as a challenge, he were to try to accept and float past the reactions that had been upsetting him and try to do his best as calmly as he could, realising that to expect more from himself in his present sensitised state would be asking the impossible. I explained the meaning of 'float' and its importance in desensitisation, and said that his slogan should be 'Float. Don't fight!'

His first experience on returning to hospital had been gruelling. He had been obliged to give an anaesthetic for a hysterectomy and in his condition this seemed particularly difficult. To make matters worse, the surgeon, scalpel in hand, had turned to him and said, 'I suppose, young man, you know that this woman has a weak heart?' The young man was so tense with fear he was on the verge of laying down his tools, when he remembered 'floating'. He knew that, in normal conditions, he could give a good anaesthetic so, reminding himself that he was being put off by no more than an obstructive thought, he released the thought to the best of his ability (helped by the idea of floating) and continued.

Had this man been subjected to months of analytical treatment searching for the cause of presumed personality inadequacy, he would have possibly become more introspective, self-conscious and critical of his efforts, and may have finally given up work at the hospital. As it was, he recovered while at his work.

I do not advise all who suffer from an anxiety state to stay at their posts, especially if they are responsible ones. Each person's capacity to cope with stress must be assessed and it is sometimes wiser to leave work temporarily. However, I must be convinced that such a drastic decision is necessary. Leaving work can be a drastic decision, because the person concerned can not only quickly lose confidence, but may be faced with idleness – his most formidable enemy. He may be at the stage where the tie between thought and emotion is so upsettingly close that idleness is torture and occupation an urgent must.

Failure of Integration

I have seen some young people who, since early youth, have had so much probing, analysis, for causes of what was considered to be unorthodox behaviour (perhaps no more than bed-wetting prolonged beyond the normal age, or reluctance to attend school) that much of the youth that should have been spent in ordinary living has been spent in psychotherapy, and perhaps part of the time in a psychiatric ward. Some of these people failed to develop an identity for themselves. As one young woman put it, 'I feel mentally dismembered, in limbo, a nothing.' She had been treated for years for post-rape trauma.

Integration for such a person comes from action, from encouragement to take part in ordinary living, not from continually questioning, probing inward into what may have become a human wilderness. It comes from doing now what he should have been doing during those years 'in psychotherapy' – living with ordinary people until he gradually feels part of normal living. At first he may feel so strange, self-conscious, unreal, it may seem to him that he is trying to mix with people from another planet. If he accepts this as an inevitable result of his past environment and is prepared to go through the misery of feeling unreal, self-conscious, uninteresting, perhaps even boring (not having lived enough in a normal world he may have little ordinary conversation), he, in my opinion, has a better chance of becoming integrated than if his disintegration is continually stressed and discussed.

At first the patient may not believe that having so little

analytical therapy will cure him. However, he soon learns that he needs much explanation and encouragement from his therapist during his early efforts at normal socialising, especially when trying to hold down a job. His shyness and sensitivity make him an easy target for any sadistic fellow worker and, unfortunately, there always seems to be one.

It is especially difficult for a person in his middle or late twenties who, having lost a youth that should have been spent in normal occupation, must now either begin to study or do unskilled work. He has, perhaps, had no practice at disciplining himself to study. Concentrating is especially difficult. There is so much to distract him. He is haunted by memory, lack of confidence and the shadow of having to return to a psychiatric hospital should he fail. Failure for him is particularly disastrous. It may mean being thrust back into idleness, into his old fears, problems, or it means trying to rise again, each time with lessened hope of success. Failure in such people needs the therapist's energetic help.

Just as confidence returns with desensitisation and understanding, reintegration follows the return of confidence. The sufferer needs to understand and accept a feeling of disintegration without being afraid of, or bewildered by, it. An understanding of sensitisation such as I have tried to give here, and then its acceptance, helps to restore inner harmony.

It may be thought that I stress acceptance too much. I cannot stress it enough. I have seen it cure so many. Indeed, I HAVE NOT SEEN IT FAIL. A critic might think, 'Of course a patient will recover if he accepts his nervous symptoms without fear! Persuading him to accept is the difficulty!' True, and this is why I stress the need for the therapist's special understanding and his adequate explanation to the patient. The therapist's ability to give explanations that the patient recognises are correct is the best advocate for acceptance. When a therapist tells a happily married agoraphobic woman that she avoids going into the street alone to protect herself against a subconscious wish to be a prostitute (as the woman in Chapter 8, agoraphobic for 28 years, had been told) and when she knows that she is simply afraid of having an attack of panic, weakness and so on when out by herself, it would be difficult for that therapist to convince that woman of anything. Indeed, that particular woman had had five analysts over 28 years, each giving a different explanation for her agoraphobia, and was finally cured by explanation of sensitisation and practical help (she describes part of her story in Chapter 8). Once more I stress that acceptance must be based on the patient's understanding sensitisation and knowing how to desensitise himself.

(7)   DEPRESSION

I discuss here the help one can give a depressed person apart from the use of orthodox treatment: antidepressants, electroconvulsive therapy, changing a life pattern and so on. For some people orthodox treatment is mandatory, but I have seen others lose a habit of depression by simply acting on the advice given below, even without the help of medication.

In this discussion, I group patients into (1) those with recurring bouts of depression who are not otherwise nervously disturbed and (2) those whose depression is part of an anxiety state.

(1)   Recurring Depression Uncomplicated by Other Nervous Disturbance

People with a habit of recurring depression respond so

quickly to an even mildly depressing atmosphere that they may but see lowering clouds at dusk to feel their spirits sink. As a rule their attention is distracted and they recover. However, if they have a few such experiences in quick succession, they begin to fear that one of their bouts is on its way. They become apprehensive, afraid. There is nothing quite so depressing as the thought of approaching depression, except the arrival of depression itself. The added strain of apprehension and fear drains their emotional reserves still further and makes depression more likely to descend.

The mistakes begin; mistakes that come from first fighting the thought of approaching depression and then from trying to fight depression once it has arrived. Take a housewife who suffers in this way. I choose a woman rather than a man because her life at home is more conducive to depression. I also choose a woman who is subjected to fairly severe bouts of depression, so that their lurking shadow is never far away.

First, this woman so dreads depression that when she feels one of her bouts approaching she rushes through her work, trying to fill each moment, so that she will have no time to think about the hovering cloud. The fight has begun. When the work is finished, she is so afraid to be alone with her thoughts, feelings, that she is off visiting one friend after another, or to the cinema, supermarket. While out, she watches herself anxiously, wondering, 'Is it still there? Will it come back when I get home?' *The best way to remember is to try too hard to forget.* So by feverishly trying to ward off depression, she may only succeed in emphasising it.

Agitated rushing is tiring. She becomes depleted, tense. Putting on an act before the family is also a strain, so the tension mounts until she finally becomes sensitised. Once sensitised, the fear she feels when she thinks of approaching depression becomes more acute. She feels this spasm of fear in the pit of her stomach, where she feels the feeling of depression. There may be so little to choose between the two feelings – fear and depression – that, as the fear mounts, she translates this into depression and is finally convinced that one of her bouts has arrived.

At this point she despairs and despair is the finishing touch. She has only to feel one flash of utter despair to admit to herself and her family that she really is depressed. Now comes the barrage of advice: 'Pull yourself together!', 'Snap out of it!', 'Fight it, Mother!' As if she hasn't been fighting it for days and getting only more deeply enmeshed. However, she starts again on the old routine, rushing, fighting, trying to 'rise above it'. She takes anti-depressants each morning to help pick herself up and tranquillisers in the afternoon to prepare her for the evening rush.

While out visiting she may forget the depression and feel almost normal, but when she thinks of it again her heart sinks immediately. The fight seems hopeless. What is the use of forgetting, when remembering brings such a painful shock! She may return home more depressed and discouraged than when she set out. At times she may start for home feeling good, only to find that the mere sight of the house throws her into despair. When so easily cast down it is difficult to remember that, in the past, depression always lifted. With each new bout there is always the fear that this one will stay.

However, emotional reserves can replenish themselves even during depression and this woman will, one morning, despite herself, probably waken to find less foreboding, more interest. From past experience she knows that depression is on its way out at last. She then fears it less, becomes less tense and is even prepared to wait patiently for it to pass.

This is a story of mismanagement that not only establishes bouts of recurring depression, but also prolongs them. Change, interesting occupation, company, are well-known prescriptions for depression. However, most people, for practical reasons, must recover in their usual routine, especially a housewife.

When a woman (or man) first feels that sinking feeling, she should try to have the courage to let it come and not run blindly from the thought of it. She should relax toward it, not tense against it, and she should try to understand that it is fostered by habit and memory and encouraged by emotional, and perhaps mental, tiredness. She should continue to work *at a steady pace* – her usual pace – not be afraid to think of herself and, above all, not be afraid to think of depression. By all means she should take every opportunity to help cheer herself, but she must do this *at a steady pace*. If she accepts that her battery of emotions is flat, that her spirits will swing up one minute and down the next for some time yet, her acceptance will cushion the shock of remembering the 'state she is in' and protect her emotions from her own onslaught upon them. This alone gives her body a chance to heal.

It takes courage to accept depression and be prepared to relax toward it, to work with it, and not seek salvation in tiring distraction. However, to face, accept and keep working at a steady pace with as little fear as possible can finally cure depression in many people without the use of anti-depressants. This treatment by willing acceptance may take longer than treatment by anti-depressants, but the confidence in self-management it brings is more desirable than reliance on drugs which may not only bring dependence but may not always cure the depression. I have taught many people, especially housewives, to cope with bouts of recurring depression in this way.

(2) *Depression in the Nervously Ill*

So far I have been talking about a woman with a habit of recurring bouts of depression. Depression in a nervously ill woman (or man) is more complicated, because it is often based on the physical depletion that may follow continuous anxiety. There may still be a desire to do things and yet a feeling of physical inability to get started; or there may be no desire to do anything. Sometimes desire may be fleeting and this, added to the strain of the nervous illness, may make life seem unendurable. It has been said that many nervously ill people could recover if they wished. When a woman (or man) is depleted, recovery may seem so far beyond her reach that she may lose heart and it may appear that she doesn't want to make the effort. Making an appointment a few days ahead seems too much. To accept an invitation for Wednesday week seems more like a threat than a promise of enjoyment. The desire to go comes only in flashes, if it comes at all. A week of procrastination brings further depletion, until she can hardly count on one positive flash of desire to go, so on Tuesday evening yet another ingenious excuse will be offered to cancel the appointment. Had the friend said, 'Come today!' the sufferer would have had a chance of mustering courage on the spur of the moment. Contemplation, as usual, is the killer. This is why planning ahead demands too much from a depleted person.

Depression is one of the most discouraging experiences in nervous illness. Unfortunately it can have such an effect on the other members of the family that joy in living may be dampened for them too. A despairing mother will say,

'Doctor, what am I to say to my daughter? Everything I do or say seems wrong!' Unfortunately, the family rarely helps the sufferer in the right way. They are likely to implore her to seek diversion – a visit here, a game of cards there, an outing in the car. She may return only temporarily helped or more discouraged than when she went out.

Curing nervous depression may take some months and expecting quick results by trying to pull or push the sufferer toward recovery will not help. If the helpers, as well as the victim, can see depression as *a state of depletion* and understand that curing will take time because a definite repletion must take place, hope and patience come into the picture.

Also, as a depressed woman (or man) recovers, it is sometimes difficult for her to know how much 'not wanting to' has become a lazy habit and how much is genuinely due to remaining depletion. Extreme depletion brings such definite symptoms that it is readily recognised as a physical state; however, as depletion eases and depression lifts, while one attempts the obvious, more interesting things readily enough, the chores most of us put off at any time still lack interest. Here the sufferer's reluctance is no more than normal dislike exaggerated. Everything cannot suddenly be interesting. A patient should be taught that, while coming out of nervous depletion, coping with the usual uninteresting tasks is especially difficult, but must be done so that a level can be reached where ordinary living becomes worthwhile.

(3) *Morning Depression*

It is strange how the morning has the disconcerting habit of disregarding improvement of the previous day. Depressed people, whether nervously ill or not, are disappointed if, after retiring hopeful, even cheerful, they wake the next morning to find the same heart of lead. To cope, the sufferer should rise on waking, have a shower, cup of tea, even switch on the radio. This is not fighting depression. This is sensible. The patient should be told how in the early morning metabolic rate is at its lowest and how rising on waking helps raise it, so that even if she must return to bed until the family rises, depression may not seem so overwhelming. Of course, if the sufferer is awake in the very early hours, it becomes a problem to decide whether to take a tranquilliser or not. Those long hours before the family stirs may stretch ahead interminably; so, for a patient in this predicament, I usually prescribe a mild sedative.

Changing bedrooms, or even the position of the bed, helps. At least the sufferer should place the bed where she is not forced to see the same pattern of things each morning when she wakes to remind her of all the other mornings of suffering and so be dragged into the quagmire of despair before she has time to orientate herself toward her new approach.

It takes courage to relax in, and go toward, depression, not tense against it in fear, not try to fight a way out of it, but to work with it at a steady pace; and yet, this approach, once mastered, can be surprisingly successful.

Whenever possible I use the word depletion rather than depression, and am gratified by the encouraging effect on the patient. She (or he) feels that she can do something about depletion, whereas the sound of depression has a ring of finality, carries threat of an onerous battle to be fought.

Once more I stress that these experiences, indecision, suggestibility and so on (which are so often grouped together as 'nervous breakdown') can follow no more than sensitisation and its resulting bewilderment and fear and to seek deep-seated causes in some patients is to hinder recovery.

CHAPTER SEVEN

First Steps to Recovery from Agoraphobia

After talking to his therapist, the agoraphobic patient may be inspired to practise travelling on his own yet may be afraid to take the first steps. He may think (1) that he has been ill for so long, he is beyond help; or (2) that he has tried so many different ways to recover in the past that trying again is too difficult; or (3) that although he understands and suspects the advice would work, he panics so easily, he wilts before each blast; or (4) that he feels so emotionally spent he may shrink from the vista of effort those first steps open up before him.

(1)   HE THINKS HE HAS BEEN ILL TOO LONG TO RECOVER

The patient should understand that no outside force is making him agoraphobic; that his body is simply responding to the way he thinks; that the symptoms of sensitisation, although alarming, are no more than a registration of sensation by nerves. I even use the word 'superficial' when describing them and the use of this simple word alone cured one patient. He should also understand that his nerves can be desensitised and that they hold no grudge against him for being ill, however long. A long span of illness means mainly that the habit of illness is strongly entrenched and has given much time for the collection of discouraging memories.

Also, while a patient may find peace and understanding when with his therapist, his tired mind easily forgets the advice given, and finding the courage to take the first steps on his own may seem too difficult. Recordings again help. I make such a recording for use on a portable cassette player (the script of this recording, 'Moving Toward Freedom', is in Chapter 12). Just as the nervous person has bombarded himself with defeatist suggestions for so long, he can now, with a recording, substitute a doctor's encouraging advice, while actually venturing out.

(2)   HE DOES NOT TRUST HIMSELF

It matters only that the patient understands the advice given and is willing to trust it. He should be taught that however big a coward he may think himself, however little he may trust himself, the advice will still work. His body will cure itself *if he stands out of its way* by adding as little second-fear as possible.

(3)   HE UNDERSTANDS, BUT FEAR FLASHES SO FIERCELY, HE
       WILTS BEFORE IT

He will probably have to accept much second-fear for the time being. When panic strikes, he may believe that he cannot think at all, so remembering quickly enough to accept flashing panic may seem impossible. It should be pointed out to him that, if he watches himself closely, he will discover that he does think, if only the wrong thoughts ('Let me out of here, quickly!'). To teach a patient a practical way to take his fears, I press my hand against his chest and ask him to move against the pressure. As he strains forward I point out that this is the tense way he has been trying to go forward. I then ask him to stretch out his arms and move them as if swimming breaststroke in deep water. I can usually feel some tension relax immediately. I explain that this is how I want him to take his panic – as if swimming in deep water. Thinking of this relaxed movement gives him something positive to do at a critical moment, instead of withdrawing blindly, tensely, in defeat.

An alternative is to instruct the patient to take a deep breath and let it out slowly. Some nervously ill people dislike the thought of water. An occasional agoraphobic will avoid taking a bath because he is afraid of having a turn while naked – quick escape is difficult.

(4)   HE THINKS HE HASN'T THE STRENGTH TO TAKE THE
        FIRST STEP

I visited a woman who, 'exhausted' by her nervous illness, had been more or less confined to a couch for months. She thought she was too weak to stand for long. I urged her to begin painting the back verandah. To her own surprise, she began. A few days later she was painting with interest and hardly noticed the chair placed strategically nearby. Much nervous weakness is based on loss of confidence in what the sufferer thinks his body can do. Because a doctor said she could paint the verandah, that woman gained enough confidence to try. I explained that the weakness of nervous illness is not caused by muscular disease and that muscles grow strong only if used.

A therapist should encourage a patient to take those first steps however long he may have been ill, however much he may distrust himself, however tired he may think himself and, above all, however afraid he may be. I try to encourage the patient to make some effort when he feels least like making it. He gets more confidence from coping with a situation when he feels at his worst, than by waiting for an auspicious moment. He should learn to wait on no mood.

THOSE FIRST STEPS

The first faltering steps (and they are faltering, almost like a child's) should never be taken quickly. A moderate pace gives time to remember the right attitude, time to understand that the sufferer is frightening himself. Speed encourages adding second-fear; it increases tension, agitation, sensitisation; it means running away not facing, although the agoraphobic may be heading in a forward direction away from home. Panic can be defeated only by those who take time to cope with it.

The agoraphobic battling his way alone down the street should not try to keep his mind off himself. Some say they try to distract themselves by counting aloud and have counted hundreds between their front gate and the pillar-box. Such a person could hardly not notice how he feels. He has been noticing his reactions so consistently for so long that sudden unawareness would be a miracle and yet he expects this from himself and despairs unnecessarily when he finds his thoughts turned on himself, his symptoms. He should understand that inward-thinking is natural in the circumstances.

The agoraphobic should go out *prepared to think continually of himself* and to have many, if not all, the familiar symptoms and fears. He should go forward toward them as willingly as possible and at the same time try to be impressed by them as little as possible (not easy!). He has been misled by physical feelings of no great medical importance for such a long time. To be unimpressed by them, he must be taught how to cope with them and not be left to try to 'get used to them'. He must also be taught that *his sensitised body is functioning normally in the circumstances of the fear and tension he is creating for it* and that, because his nerves have been conditioned to bring heightened responses, acceptance will not perform miracles overnight. It may be the first time in years that he is trying to go out by himself, so being anxiously on guard must be expected and accepted and any stress symptoms that occur must not be regarded as sick reactions but understood as normal in the circumstances of his apprehension.

Also, each person must be prepared to recover at his own pace. Slow recovery has advantages; it gives repeated opportunity to practise the right way, until the right reaction becomes routine.

RIGHT REACTION-READINESS

Right reaction-readiness means that an agoraphobic has prepared himself by practice, either in fantasy or in vivo, to meet stressful situations often enough to have established the right approach as a habit. In the early stages of recovery, the sufferer remembers past failures so vividly, and the dreaded symptoms that accompanied them stand out so clearly, that unwittingly he is in a state of wrong reaction-readiness whenever he attempts to take those first steps.

Right reaction-readiness can be practised at home. It will not only prepare the agoraphobic to move away from home, but it will also prepare him to face other personal difficulties.

To practise right reaction-readiness at home, the patient should sit as comfortably as possible and imagine himself in one of the situations he most dreads – for example, waiting to board a bus. As the imaginary bus approaches, he should try to feel the same misgivings he would feel if actually at the bus-stop; try to make the reactions as severe as he can and at the same time try to stay as relaxed as possible. Some therapists say relaxation is not important to these people, that the same results are achieved if they are tense. This may be so for the technique called 'flooding', when the patient may even be encouraged to be tense, the objective being to show himself that he can pass through the worst symptoms, the greatest panic, and come to no harm. Flooding has its merits for some, but terrifies others. I prefer to teach the patient how to pass through the worst moment until he knows he can cope with it. However, I do encourage a patient to let panic do its worst, if necessary, to let it 'burn the roots of his hair!', but, I stress once more, I teach him how to go through the moment when his hair is burning.

If the patient wearies of hearing the word 'accept', one can substitute the expression 'reacting freely', which means to give full range to his nervous sensations and reactions, to let them all come. Many a nervously ill person fears that by doing this the feelings will be so overpowering that he will be immobilised by them. The word 'freely' saves him. It releases tension, encourages action and eventually desensitises.

Different words, phrases, have different effects on people. Reacting freely is descriptive; it tells its own story. A patient said recently that the phrase that helped her most was 'You have been bluffed by physical feelings;' another said that her particular, helpful phrase was 'Practise, don't test', and yet another woman was cured by 'The symptoms are superficial'.

The patient entering a bus in fantasy should choose a seat at the front, even imagine himself groping for the fare while the conductor waits impatiently. Once settled in his imaginary seat, he can remind himself that he cannot leave the bus in a hurry, can imagine any emergency (perhaps the bus breaking down and having to change buses) at the same time reminding himself of what he should do. He should put this into words. The more he practises at home, the more readily the right reaction will come when he puts himself into the real situation.

One woman wrote, 'I can't remember your advice quickly enough to freewheel past panic and other nervous symptoms.' The practice just described would help her, but I would prefer that she were not so anxious to free-wheel past panic. This is too much like trying to switch panic off. Because of her long-established wrong reaction-readiness, this woman asks herself a physiological impossibility at this stage of her illness. *Panic will cease to come only when it, and other nervous symptoms, switch themselves off because their coming no longer matters.* When that woman has learnt to pass through the symptoms the right way, they will no longer overwhelm her. True avoidance becomes automatic and there will no longer be a struggle to remember the right advice.

Also, when the agoraphobic travels, he should try to loosen the tense hold on home; try to cut the tie between home and himself; try to move forward in thought and, if in a vehicle, to move forward with it.

The person is rare indeed who always copes with panic the right way in the early stages of recovery. In the beginning, practising moving away from home makes most people more sensitised and more tired than when remaining in the safety of their house. When willing to put himself in the front line of battle, the agoraphobic could have more panic than he has had for a long time past, so that he may at this stage need tranquillisation, but never enough to deaden all nervous reaction. He must feel some fear and its effects to be able to practise coping with it.

Because of the increased sensitisation during the early efforts, some agoraphobics lose heart. On the other hand, the person who has once glimpsed what acceptance can achieve may become so dedicated to it that he may be afraid to let one day pass without practising for fear of losing his gain of the previous day. He must be taught to accept halts in recovery. To sometimes refresh without making effort is necessary.

When a patient fails, he should be taught that it is because he *did* rush to get it over; *did* withdraw in fear; *did* try to sit on panic; *did* try to switch panic off; *did* add too much second-fear; or was over-tired, over-sensitised with so much endeavour that he became frightened by the increased intensity of his reactions at a time when he thought he should be feeling better. Maybe he listened to the little voice always ready to discourage, the voice that says, 'Others can do it, but not you!' That voice is so ready to discourage that the patient should learn to recognise it, expect it, and practise floating past it.

He should try to recognise the difference between practising and testing. If he went round the park well last week, he should not try to do as well this week and then be disappointed if he fails. Desire to do as well the second time could mean beginning the second journey more apprehensively than the first, so that only minor stress could throw him into panic and disappointment. *He should practise, not test.* The way to recovery is tricky and drugs will not compensate for a lack of understanding among patients or therapists of the many obstacles in the way. Adequate explanation is still the best treatment, because without it the sufferer takes every baffling turn and twist in his illness seriously.

Acceptance through understanding not only brings relief from sensitisation, it also relieves the sufferer from asking himself the everlasting 'Why?', so mental fatigue lifts and a refreshed mind, no longer blinkered by one point of view, can bring troublesome situations into better perspective.

Once more I stress that the patient should watch for the moment of recoil and go right through it. One hundred per cent acceptance is the answer, not 99 per cent.

An aeroplane pilot explained that the same principle held in aeronautics. When a plane is going into a fall, one of the hardest lessons for a beginner to learn is to point the plane into the direction of the fall. To go this way is to flatten out and recover. To dip the wings in the opposite direction can be catastrophic.

It is important that the patient should not be put off by the places or experiences he fears. These are his salvation because they are his practising ground and recovery, the final establishment of the right attitude, lies in them.

The patient may shrink from the demands that the thought of recovery may bring. He imagines meeting them as he now feels – a kaleidoscope of feelings. But recovery brings its own change, renewed strength and interest. The patient must go forward with trust in this change and in the gradual ability to cope that it brings. It is the gradualness that makes all possible, but it is also this gradualness that is so difficult to bear because it is so frustrating and allows so much time for contemplation. Only the confidence and understanding that comes from repeated doing eventually takes the fear out of contemplation. And, as already stressed, the patient should learn to wait on no mood. It is the sitting, waiting, hat and coat on, hands clenched, contemplating moving that is so devastating. Salvation lies in repeated doing.

Some therapists encourage patients to travel only as far as they can without panicking and to return immediately if the panic starts. In this way they hope to desensitise the patient. I have not met one patient cured by this approach. Some have been made worse, because of increased awareness of a necessity to avoid panic. While such therapists put much conscientious effort into helping their patients, they would get more gratifying results were they to teach them how to cope with panic, rather than avoid it.

CHAPTER EIGHT

Obstacles to Recovery

Each of these articles gives insight into the patient's point of view, reaction, when in certain adverse situations common to those struggling to recover from an anxiety state, especially an anxiety state accompanied by agoraphobia.

(1)   THE SMALL COFFEE SHOP

A letter from America:

'My general practitioner is pleased with what I have done. He saw me through 12 years of not being able to do anything. He felt helpless as I could not follow his advice. I was too terrified to try. Then I learnt about sensitisation and acceptance and this got me going at last.

'I have had severe setbacks. At one time I thought I was back at my very worst. But I pulled out. I have a feeling of

"What now?", as if maybe I'm cured, although I know I'm not, as you will see as you read on. I don't get the elated feeling I used to get when I did things. Maybe I feel no challenge.

'I've been working for the first time in 22 years. I think I'm almost at a cured point. Maybe I'm normal and don't recognise it. After being anxious for 12 years, perhaps I've forgotten what it's like to feel normal.

'For example, this is one of my frustrating hang-ups. After going thru [*sic*] a week of hell anticipating a hockey game, *the* night came and I went without any of the fearful feelings I'd been having. Crowds bother me as a rule, but there were 30 thousand people at that game and, except for a slight giddiness, I had no anxious feelings. I was happy, but I did not have the elated feeling I thought I should have had.

'I can do this [the hockey match] and yet in a small coffee shop I can still have an awful time. There are other small things left I can't do. This is what puzzles me. I don't seem able to handle the coffee shops. I've been practicing for three months, at least once a week. I've tried different shops in different areas, but always have a bad time. I have not tried having dinner out, as I was hoping to do this step by step, starting with the coffee shop. I have said to panic, "Come and do your worst!" but I'm always glad to get away. Other agoraphobics say the same thing. I'm wondering if making the effort and going all the way into a crowded restaurant would help me cope with the small shops?'

Elation, the motivator in early stages in recovery, must give way to calm satisfaction as the agoraphobic becomes used to accomplishment. Such an acute emotion as elation is rare at any time. So, when no longer elated, the agoraphobic is beginning to feel like other people. Although this woman appreciates this, she hankers after that wonderful feeling, elation.

At this point in recovery, she will anticipate fearfully before any difficult undertaking, because she has done so for so many years, and has not managed well often enough yet to dull the edge of memory – anxious anticipation is her habit.

When *the* night arrived, she felt a certain relief from strain because the waiting was over, so she felt more relaxed. Because she was more relaxed, she could now concentrate on remembering the previous recent occasions when she managed well and this encouragement carried her off to the hockey match. That week of dreadful anticipation was *normal in the circumstances*, not a hang-up. It may be a year or more before she can take any challenging outing without some anxious anticipation; this is one of the last phases of agoraphobia to lift.

Not being able to cope with a small coffee shop illustrates the mistake of trying to cope with a special situation and not with fear itself. This woman asks if doing a big thing (sitting in a crowded restaurant) would make sitting in a small shop easier. It might, but she is much more likely to approach the coffee shop in such a state of 'Will I be able to do it now?' that she would be more likely to be apprehensive, agitated, before she even reached there. So much depends on attitude and when one is susceptible to flashing panic, the right attitude is difficult to maintain; the old flash knows its way round every corner. In those small shops she has suffered so much that the memory of suffering is always waiting for her. As long as she thinks in terms of *a place to cope with*, she could remain afraid of the small shops, however well she managed in a crowded restaurant. In the coffee shop she still withdraws in fear. Although she says, 'Come and do your worst!' she means

'Come and get it over, so that I can get out of here as quickly as possible, and when you do your worst, please don't be too severe!'

This is not good enough. She must learn to regard a small coffee shop as a place where she has an opportunity to practise facing and coping with panic and other nervous feelings, until they no longer matter. *It is always the moment she must cope with, not the place.*

(2) AN AGORAPHOBIC FOR 28 YEARS DESCRIBES
     HER GRADUAL RECOVERY

'When I first read about sensitisation, I thought that here at last was an understanding of how to cope with my illness. The more I studied the more the explanation seemed right.

'I agreed that curing the state I was in was the important thing and not trying to find an original cause. I never could understand how finding a cause hidden beneath 28 years of suffering could help my agoraphobia now. To take myself in my own hands, regardless of the past, and not look for outside help to make recovery easy was a challenge I knew I must face at last, if I wished to recover. For the past 15 years, except for entering local small shops, I had gone nowhere without being accompanied by my children's nurse and if I had to go on a journey of any length, I always took a doctor with me. I was a severe, chronic agoraphobic.

'However, I had become so desperate that I finally decided to try the basic theory of facing, accepting, floating and letting time pass. I must say the thought of letting more time pass filled me with dismay, as half my life had gone in illness. However, I took off with some enthusiasm and achieved minor successes in moving about which I had not made in years. Surely, I thought, there must be more to recovery than taking off in a flash this way? I soon learned that for me there was because, before long, the early elation passed and I was back where I had started.

'For weeks this cycle repeated itself – minor successes followed by fatigue and no real feeling of growing confidence. Each adventure seemed too great an ordeal. However, I could not forget the glimpse of success I had had earlier. I had touched something I was unable to grasp, *but I had touched it!*

'I realised that although some could go out immediately and not look back, others would find facing, accepting, floating and letting time pass very difficult. I had to accept that I was one of these. I remembered the words, "Each recovers in his own time, accept even that." Realising that this method would work for me only if I was ready to accept it fully and let the cure come from inside myself in its own time, I finally accepted the time involved.

'It was hard to think cure had to come from me for I had always hoped for it from an outside source, and yet, however hard it was to work by myself, a little voice inside me kept niggling, making me keep on course. On one occasion, after I had managed to travel for some distance from home, everything seemed to recede. I felt lost, incapable of even asking someone for help. This feeling of recession was worse than panic. However, I thought I must meet it the same way as panic – wait, take it slowly. Finally I was able to hail a taxi.

'I managed successfully one day and failed the next. I became desperate when I heard of fellow sufferers who were making quicker progress than I. I suspected I might not have what it took to stay in the race.

'Sometimes my illness seemed a safer way of life; at least I knew where I stood and this seemed better than being a perpetual emotional yo-yo, better one day, worse the next.

But once I had started, I could not give up.

'A few days later I drove around Hyde Park on my own. Panic after panic flashed. When I returned, spent and upset, I nearly vomited. This, I decided, was my last attempt. I would stop the whole thing now! But somehow I didn't feel as relieved as I had expected. That little voice kept niggling, "Where have you gone wrong? Why have you failed?" Trembling, because I suspected that that wretched voice would make me try to do the journey again, I analysed where I had made mistakes and suddenly knew I had accepted nothing. I had tried to get through the journey at the fastest possible speed and had withdrawn from panic by trying to blast my way through it. My one thought had been to get home as quickly as possible. I decided to drive round the park again and this time to make success out of failure. I set off very, very slowly, ready to meet panic when it came. On that first journey I knew I had added so much second-fear. At my special panic-place, I slowed down almost to a crawl. Of course I panicked, but I saw it right through and kept going forward slowly, but willingly, with the car. Three times I repeated the journey and I did not panic again. I saw at last that recovery would begin to work only through experience and that this was why it must take time.

'I now became almost obsessional in my desire to experiment with myself. I was afraid to let one day pass without doing something new. I thought that if I did, I would lose the progress I had made. This was a mistake, because it made me more tired. I was trying too hard. I learned to take even this aspect of recovery more sensibly.

'In spite of now feeling I'm on the right track, I'm sometimes nervier than when in the shelter of my agoraphobia. But I know that this is because I am meeting situations I have avoided for years. It is obvious that beginning to recover may bring increased sensitisation and this makes one feel as if no progress has been made. However, when I repeat some of the earlier steps, I find them surprisingly easy. The other day I found entering a store alone effortless. Formerly I had done so at great cost. This brought hope.

'Recovery sometimes makes me feel unreal. For more than 20 years illness has been my reality. I suppose it is only natural these new experiences should feel strange. I do understand that only when accomplishment is no longer a novelty will my changed way of life begin to feel real. Setback, exhaustion, depression, panic all seem part of failure, yet I have learned that I cannot go forward without them. This is a hard lesson because it is not easy to put oneself voluntarily into situations that may bring these experiences. Although I'm only at the beginning of the road, I have had those moments of glimpsing recovery which have brought me such hope that I feel that to turn back now would be impossible and I fear going forward less.

'I am now trying to work without props. I used to think I could always telephone home and someone would come. Now I go off when no one is home. Recently, with as little contemplation as possible, I went 15 miles by car. It was a great moment. It was not easy, and three days later I made a mess of the same journey. But I have learned that I cannot stay happy when I fail. I must go again and correct my mistakes. As Dr Weekes explains, recovery lies in repeated doing, until enough achievement replaces defeatist contemplation. I still have my full share of that, especially at night, when, head on pillow, it all seems impossible. But the next day somehow I'm at it again, and once I'm in the car, the doing takes over. I know that, for complete recovery, the day must come when the cord of dependence between myself and outside support must be completely cut. This is what I'm working at now.'

Last summer brought much domestic strain on this woman, but she has been able to consolidate the progress she made. She can now drive alone to the golf-course, seven miles away, and play all day without having the children's nurse in the neighbourhood. She recently drove 200 miles and stayed overnight at a country hotel after attending her son's school concert at night. She also goes to cinemas, concerts and into shops either alone or with her children and when she remembers agoraphobia it is to think how once she could not do these things.

(3) A DAY IN THE LIFE OF A NERVOUSLY ILL HOUSEWIFE

Since the majority of my patients have been housewives, many alone all day, I will describe a routine day in the life of such a woman choosing an agoraphobic who suffers at home as well as away from home and will show how she holds back recovery. The situation of the nervously ill spinster, bachelor or married man who struggles to work each day is much the same; at least it is not difficult to substitute their situation for hers and to apply the same advice to it.

Waking Up

When a nervously ill housewife wakes in the morning, realisation that she must face another day may strike before she opens her eyes. The thought brings anguish, stress. As she wakes further and remembers some threatening duty of the day – perhaps a school concert in the evening – more anguish follows, until the exaggerated symptoms of stress she dreads appear and finally merge into one long inner churning – a disappointing, tiring start to the day.

After further panic, with her resistance already lowered by months, or years, of suffering, she may feel exhausted, depressed. The energy she gained from her night's rest has been almost depleted by nervous reaction to her own thoughts, before she even tries to get out of bed. Her limbs may feel so leaden that she may feel incapable of moving; however, necessity finally forces her to rise and 'point the body' (as one woman expressed it) at the day's work.

As she fumbles under the bed for her slippers, repetition of stooping and groping brings back the memory of countless mornings when she has done the same, feeling as she feels now. Trapped by memory, her thoughts become all despair and since her body is at the mercy of her thoughts she feels 'worse than ever'. She has made the mistake of making memory part of the day's burden.

When the noise of the family's departure is stilled by the final closure of the front door, the sudden silence seems more overpowering than the noise. At least noise meant someone was there – a prop to divert her attention. Now all attention is directed toward herself. The last thing she wants is to have her mind on herself and her illness, and yet she knows this is what she will have all day. There seems no way out for her. Her heart thumps at the thought. More anguish. She pours herself a cup of tea before facing the dishes in the sink and, while she drinks, she thinks how hopeless it is, how futile to imagine she can possibly recover, when she can hardly find the strength or courage to face one day.

She has been turning in a circle of defeat like the blind-folded ass that drags the millstone – memory of past suffering and the anticipated suffering of the day ahead bring despair . . . despair brings stress . . . stress brings even more acutely sensitised feelings . . . and these lead to more despair.

This pattern is repeated in so many of the day's activities. She may not leave the house to go shopping until mid-morning and, between waking and setting off, she gives herself spasms of panic whenever she thinks of the outing to come. Hours of intermittent panic would weaken even a strong man, so by the time mid-morning comes she feels weak, light-headed, giddy. She has been expecting and dreading this. It is one reason why she doesn't want to go out alone. She had hoped today might be different, but once again she will be forced to send the children shopping when they return from school.

At the thought of school, her heart misses a beat. How will she manage the school meeting that evening, when she feels so weak already? And what if they ask her to look at the children's paintings in the hot, crowded classroom. The school function means half an hour under the drier at the hairdresser's! More anguish.

So, there she is. To every situation, and yet such ordinary situations, she reacts with panic. She does not understand that her body's reactions are normal in the circumstances, that the sickness lies in their exaggeration, not in their actual occurrence. When she thinks of not going to the school function and disappointing the family yet again, she feels desperate. The tension of indecision brings on agitation, and when this happens she is utterly defeated.

She Dreams the Impossible Dream

If the nervously ill housewife expects to wake feeling well at this stage in her illness, she dreams the impossible dream. One night's sleep will not work a miracle. Yet each night when she goes to bed, she prays for just that. Her very hopes are preparing the way for disappointment the next day. If only one could say to her at night, 'Don't be disappointed, however you feel when you wake tomorrow; do not add despair and exhaust yourself still further; *try to take yourself as you find yourself.* You'll be sensitised for some time yet, so if you can only "point the body" at this stage, point it *willingly*.'

When she fumbles for her slippers, she needs special help. She should at least buy new slippers; if possible, foolish ones that make her smile. And she might try to remember not to put them under the bed each night. Breaking the chain of memories, even in such foolish ways as this, helps. To help herself further, she could change the position of the furniture in the room, especially the bed, so that on waking she does not see the same familiar pattern of things which also remind her of the many other mornings of suffering.

She would help herself during those hours of waiting to go shopping if she were to think, 'If I keep frightening myself, of course my legs will feel weak, and I'll feel giddy. It's natural, not illness. Even if my legs go weak, they can still carry me.' And if only she would add, 'Of course I'll feel awful at the hairdresser's. I've been feeling awful there for so long, I'm not going to stop feeling that way now just because I want to. I may make great strides doing other things – like going on a vacation – and still find going to the hairdresser's difficult. This doesn't mean that I'm sick again. It means only that memory is up to its tricks. I'll probably have to sit many hours at the hairdresser's thinking the right way before I break the habit of dreading being there.'

Two Kinds of Sufferers

One kind of sufferer says, 'I can't help the feelings coming. They just come. I'm not doing it to myself! I suddenly feel dreadful, when I'm not even thinking about my illness. That is what is so hard to understand!'

The other says, 'I know I'm doing this to myself but I

feel powerless to stop it! That is what is so terrible!'

There are times when nervous symptoms seem to strike for no apparent reason and are unrelated to the sufferer's occupation at the time. Past suffering has conditioned nervous reactions to come so swiftly that the slightest stimulus, unrecognised by the sufferer and beyond his direct control, may bring them. It is within his power, however, to gradually soothe this hyper-irritability by accepting these apparent out-of-the-blue attacks and by not being continually baffled and upset by them.

The person who says he is powerless to stop frightening himself must try to understand that his feeling of frightening himself is a natural outcome of his sensitised, quick response to his slightest anxious thought. As I have pointed out before, feeling, especially fear, may follow thought so closely in a sensitised person that not only do thought and feeling seem as one, but sometimes it seems as if there is no thought, only feeling. This is so confusing that the nervously ill person naturally thinks he is frightening himself and, in a sense, he is; however when he understands sensitisation and learns to desensitise himself, by acceptance and not adding second-fear, the intensity of his nervous reaction is reduced and he can then reason without so much upsetting reaction. To help himself do this he must try to look ahead and not be too impressed with the sensations, or emotions, of the moment. A long-range programme of acceptance based on understanding will reduce tension and so gradually allow him to think more calmly, even of fear itself.

(4) DIFFICULTY IN RETURNING HOME

Telling a nervously ill housewife that she may soon return home from hospital, or holiday, is not always a happy task. I am cautious when I mention going home, even to a woman who has made good progress away from home. Some wilt when given this news. The patient senses how critical the first few weeks at home may be; that she may either go forward to recovery, or relapse into illness and into a despair that she senses may be more desperate than ever, because of the tantalising glimpse of recovery she has had while away. She knows that she is returning to the same routine that may have helped to make her ill. She also knows that the family may think they have done their part doing without her, and that she, as well as they, should now be able to forget the upsetting experience. The patient understands this attitude, but fears it. She knows that her veneer of recovery is thin. Experience warns her that recovery will take time and she knows that necessity, particularly her family's necessity, may not allow her time. One of my patients was greeted at the front door with, 'Thank Heavens you're home! Now we can have some decent food at last!'

The housewife also knows that friends or relatives may put themselves out once to mind the children while she's away, but twice? Small wonder that, as time for returning home approaches, her growing apprehension may bring relapse. Unfortunately this may be interpreted by her therapist as a wish to escape into illness to avoid responsibility. This is so far from the truth that she becomes more upset.

Also, the woman improving away from home knows that much of her improvement came from having her day filled with change and occupation in the company of others and, what is more, occupation within the limits of her capacity. She fears that when she is at home occupation will certainly not be within the limits of her capacity. Before leaving hospital she may think, 'How will I react to being home? Will I slip back?' She should understand that her feelings will be mixed; she will be glad to be home one minute and frightened the next; afraid of seeing the places again where she has suffered and yet glad to be home with the people she loves, at the same time worried lest she disappoint them and becomes ill again. She should admit these feelings to herself not shy away from them, but at the same time know that none is permanent, none important. She should take with her the knowledge that reconciled acceptance of such strange feelings gradually abolishes them.

Despite resolutions, the patient's condition may deteriorate on first returning home. She may be left alone all day and the contrast with being with people while away may seem unbearable. Also, in spite of preparing herself for distressing memories around the house, actual contact with them can be so upsetting, that she may fail to distinguish between reality and memory, so, as she wanders from room to room, assailed by painful recollections, she may think, 'What's wrong! I'm no better than before I went away!'

One woman who considered herself cured telephoned joyously after a holiday to say how well she felt and that she was coming to show herself to me the next day. She arrived looking well enough, but did not seem as radiant as she had sounded on the telephone. Indeed, she wore the shadow of the old frightened look. I said, 'You were surprised to find that as soon as you sat in this familiar chair, your old fears came back?' She answered, 'They were back before that, Doctor! As soon as I put my foot on your stairs they were back! What's wrong with me?'

I said, 'You can't immediately forget the suffering associated with climbing those stairs. But understand *this is only memory* and don't be bluffed by it.' Her setback lasted about two weeks and it was necessary to telephone her several times during that period. She is completely recovered now.

Touching the stars

An agoraphobic woman, who had not left home for years, managed to cross the English Channel and holiday in Switzerland. After returning home she wrote, 'I touched the stars but I can't do it again! On returning home, my old fears flooded back all too quickly and, of course, they seem so much worse after tasting that wonderful freedom while away.'

To grasp and hold stars, there must be frequent opportunity to practise doing it and such opportunity is rare in one's own home environment. How humdrum it seems in comparison with the beauty, excitement of that successful journey in a distant land. Coming back to the familiar brings so many shocks; there is nothing more spirit-crushing than hearing the washing machine grinding away at the holiday wash, as if nothing unusual had happened.

It helps if the patient realises that the non-nervously ill person may also go through a similar experience of seeing the holiday balloon burst. Ecstasy is only ecstasy because it is short lived. So the woman who touched the stars should not lament if she cannot believe she did. She should not be surprised if, despite the experience, she feels on her return she has made no progress and may even seem unable to re-establish the progress she had made toward recovering from agoraphobia before going away. She will not lose what she has gained, *if she lets the first shock pass*, lets more time pass and does not prolong the suffering memory brings by revolting against it. How uncomfortably convincingly real feelings of the moment can be to nervously ill people.

The script of a tape recording 'Going on Holiday' (which includes a section on returning home) is included in Chapter 12.

(5) A HUSBAND'S ATTITUDE TO HIS WIFE'S AGORAPHOBIA

Although a husband may begin by sympathising with an agoraphobic wife, he may eventually become critical, desperate at the inconvenience the illness brings. The wife will struggle on, aware of the difficulties only too well and feeling guilty because of them. Contemplating taking an agoraphobic woman on holiday is especially frustrating. One minute she says she'll go; the next, she can't manage it. Reservations are made and cancelled several times. No small part of a man's frustration lies in his swinging from optimism at his wife's improvement to despair when she slips once more into a setback that makes no sense to him. She also has her share of frustration when, because of disappointment or lack of interest, her husband fails to give the co-operation she craves. She feels this acutely, because frustration, like so many of her emotions, is exagerrated by sensitisation. She may be bewildered by her antipathy toward him and think, 'What is real? My present dislike, or my old love?' Although she knows the love must be there she cannot feel it. A nervously ill person should not sigh too deeply for a family's understanding. Most sufferers follow a lonely road, hedged by misunderstanding.

A woman will say, 'When I try to explain to my husband, I can see by the look on his face that he thinks I'm crazy. It's not his fault. But I wish he wouldn't go to pieces when he sees me like this, and I wish he wouldn't think he helps me when he tries to force me to do things. It's when he forces that the tension mounts and that's what frightens me so much!' The added tension of being watched by critical eyes keeps a wife in a cycle of tension-guilt-tension.

A husband's co-operation is so important that a therapist should explain as fully to him as to his wife the meaning of sensitisation and how it can be cured. If he is reluctant to listen, tape recordings may help. The husband finds himself listening despite himself. Even critical relatives may listen from curiosity and become less critical.

If a therapist can take the trouble to help the husband understand and be patient, the husband's reward will be the grateful love of a wife who will never forget his strength and kindness in her illness; if he does not understand or help, despite the many excuses she will make for him, she will find it difficult to forget that he failed her when she needed him most, and her illness may drag on unnecessarily.

(6)   OCCUPATION

Occupation as a crutch in recovery from nervous illness has long been recognised. However, *it is essential that a nervously ill person does not throw himself into occupation because he is afraid to think of his illness.* He must have a programme for recovery which guides and supports him while he works. As well as explaining the nature of his symptoms, experiences and the four concepts (facing, accepting, floating and letting time pass) I sometimes teach a patient to imagine that his mind is divided into two parts, one part that suffers while it works and the other that accepts the suffering and looks on, almost like an overseer. I explain that the part that suffers may do so for a considerable time while waiting for recovery; however, because of the part that accepts, (the overseer), the patient is not working blindly, bewildered. When he is prepared in this way, occupation can replace painful by impersonal thought and so hasten desensitisation.

It is easier to find occupation for a man than a woman. A man may continue at his usual work, which at least means companionship and working away from home. However, if his work includes concentrating on intricate problems, mental fatigue may be a formidable obstacle and the patient may need guidance to cope with it. Usually he struggles to succeed through a barrier of loss of confidence, fear, inability to concentrate and suspicion that his brain has been damaged by his illness. I mention this because one man, an engineer, said he was near suicide for these reasons. He did not understand that a tired mind may work at a very slow pace. He recovered when he learnt to work as slowly as his tired mind demanded, and not to make an issue of solving any difficult engineering problem.

The housewife, left to make beds, wash up, sweep floors, with only tradesmen or children to talk to, has little to distract her and works automatically and in a place where she is constantly reminded of her illness. If she had her first attack of palpitations while washing up, the sink now holds special fear.

The families of most middle-aged women have either married and left home or work daily away from home, so the woman is often finished work by midday and is left with the long, lonely afternoon hours stretching ahead.

An agoraphobic woman in a severe anxiety state, who panicked at home as well as when out, described how she felt when the family had left for the day.

'A feeling sweeps over me. My face burns; my throat keeps closing. My lips are dry. I tremble. I cry and feel as though I'm going to smother. My stomach is churning. I don't want to be alone. I clench my hands, they are tense. My neck muscles are tense. My legs feel weak. My head feels tight, as though it is going to lift. I have sat at the verandah table. This is something I had been unable to do before. Before, when I have felt this turn coming on, my impulse was to rush into the garden and pace about. I now feel a little better. My husband has gone. I feel awful when he goes. I'm going to try and be sensible and go in and wash up and talk to my little dog.'

The next day, she wrote, 'I woke up and thought I must go with my husband and daughter, but they couldn't take me. Later the feeling of being alone swept over me. Tomorrow they are going early. I still feel tense but will do some housework. I will wait all day now. This is a big problem.'

This woman should never have been left alone at this stage in her illness. If leaving home temporarily, or even having company at home, is impossible, at least the therapist should, if practicable, visit the house and see the place where he is expecting his patient to recover. I had advised this woman to sit on her verandah rather than stay isolated in the dark house and she had done so conscientiously but with little good effect. I did not know, until I saw it, that the verandah was enclosed by a partition and that when seated she could not see over it.

Company is almost as important as occupation. A student recovering from an anxiety state was staying with friends in the country and was obliged to be alone during the day. He was in a state of almost compulsive, continuous introspection. However, one of the friends managed to stay home for two weeks. The mental crutch this companionship brought was beginning to lift him out of his upsetting inward-thinking when, unfortunately, the friend returned to work. The student said he was sure that if he had had company for a little longer he would have been lifted out of his habit of anxious introspection long enough to be refreshed and regain the command over his thoughts that he craved. As it was, he had to literally watch himself slip into setback and know that he could only accept it and wait for more time to pass. At least he understood his illness and the effect of mental fatigue upon it.

Rest and quiet may be mistakenly prescribed for some nervously ill people. It is sometimes easier to recover within the noisy diversions of the city than in the pressing solitude of the country; for many people, to sit and sip an ice-cream soda in a busy café, watching people coming and going, can help distract a tired mind and lift depressed spirits much more than the sound of the babbling brook.

Returning to work may be enough to cure some people if it successfully takes their mind off their problems long enough to refresh it and so lessen their exaggerated emotional reaction, so that they can face their problems less emotionally. However, returning to work is more likely to succeed if the sufferer returns with a programme for recovery to support and guide him.

Although the person recovering from nervous illness may not be as afraid as he was, he may be unable to lose a constant feeling of apprehension. This bewilders. He feels as if something terrible were about to happen and yet he knows his real trouble has passed. This is the shadow of the shadow, an emotional habit that follows months, years, of true anxiety. Time and acceptance will relieve it, but they may work so slowly that the sufferer may seek a doctor's help. She (it is usually a housewife in this predicament without the variety, change, that occupation away from home can bring) often describes herself as more 'flat' than depressed or unhappy. She is easily discouraged. She thinks, 'I'll go to town!' but when she considers bathing, dressing, catching a bus she puts off going. These people are pleased to hear that this is no more than an emotional habit, that they are not going mental, and that the habit can be cured.

Some lose the habit of carrying anxiety around by temporarily working away from home. Others must lose it in other ways.

One woman wrote that she recovered by 'nurping' (her word). By this she meant indulging herself in some small way each day; for example, if she saw violets, instead of thinking how expensive they were – as she used to – she bought them and made a point of stopping to smell and admire them during the day. In this way she gradually grew used to the feeling of happiness once more.

Occupation is a problem that must be solved for each patient. I can but emphasise its necessity for a nervously ill person. If further proof were needed, one has but to compare a patient, who works away from home, on Friday with the same person on Monday after an idle week-end. 'Week-ends kill me!' said one man.

(7)   TRANQUILLISATION

Using tranquillisers to quieten sensitisation completely not only carries the danger of drug dependence, it does little to help the patient permanently. Of the 528 agoraphobic men and women in the 1970 survey, approximately 50% were already receiving tranquillisers from their general practitioner or psychiatrist when they first began my treatment by remote direction; however, some wrote and said they were able to cut down the dose during this treatment and others said they could finally manage without medication. Some of these had been formerly told they must remain on drugs for the rest of their lives. The remaining 50% preferred to work without drugs.

I use mainly diazepam or sodium amytal. I have not, to my knowledge, had a patient addicted to barbiturates. This may be because I try to limit their use to two or three months.

Of course there is occasionally the very severely sensitised, depleted person who needs continuous sedation for a week or more. If possible, I prefer to sedate such a person in his home (with supervision, of course) rather than in hospital.

CHAPTER NINE

Coming Through Setback

Memory may recall old fears so vividly that the victim easily mistakes memory for reality and thinks he is ill again. The nervously ill person has seen those houses, those shops, those streets so often that the very sight spells weariness, illness. The therapist should understand in depth the pitfalls memory can bring if he hopes to cure his patient.

I use homely similies when possible. They relate more convincingly to the patient's illness and are easy for him to remember. For instance, when I returned home from school, my grandmother often had a batch of hot scones ready. Today, years later, when I smell hot scones, I often think 'Grandma!' almost as a reflex reaction. I point out to the patient that there is the same relationship between my flashback memory and his remembering his illness at the sight, or smell, of some place where he once suffered. I suggest that when memory flashes and symptoms return, he should think, 'It's only Grandma's scones!' Because of my books, recordings, journals, there are thousands (literally) of erstwhile agoraphobic people today walking in places they have not dared venture into for years, helped by the thought of Grandma's scones when some disturbing memory threatens to drag them into a setback.

Many people think that, as they recover, setbacks

should come less frequently and be progressively less severe and so they may, but the worst setback of all can come just before cure. The nearness of recovery makes a setback at this time especially bewildering. Also, some setbacks come with unaccountable suddenness, even when recovery seems established. One woman wrote, 'I have done well desensitising myself. I have a return of panic about once a month now; but the further apart the spells come, the less I know how to handle them. They come with a greater shock after a peaceful period. I'm so out of practice then, that for a while I forget the right advice.'

Another woman wrote, 'When in setback I walk round the house all day giving myself words, words, words; it takes quite a time to feel in charge of the situation. But this is getting better as I practise. I feel more confident each time I come through a setback and remember the way out more readily.' In other words, she is beginning to know the way out so well that she fears the way in less.

Another bewildering aspect of setback can be the surprisingly quick return of all the upsetting symptoms, almost like a chain reaction. The sufferer is tempted to think that the number of returning symptoms is a measure of the severity of the setback. I explain that if he thinks of his cousin John, the chances are he will then think of other members of the family, and that this is no more than a linkage of related memories. The symptoms of setback are the symptoms of stress. Since a setback itself brings added stress, reappearance of many stress symptoms is to be expected.

Many ask if they must always have setbacks. Setbacks no longer come only when the sufferer loses his fear of them. When no longer feared a setback may be so mild that it may dwindle into being no more than a memory of past suffering and, after a few pangs of anguish at remembering, the sufferer may then switch to being grateful for having had the experience.

If a setback seems inordinately long, the patient should beware of thinking that because it is so long it will never pass. If he examines himself, he will find that he is waiting too impatiently for it to go, that he *is* withdrawing in fear, *is* falling into the trap of trying to fight his way through it. He must give as much time to coming through a setback as it demands and not try to test himself each morning to see if he is getting better, not watch himself too anxiously. One can rarely step out of a setback quickly in the early stages of recovery. Each setback must be given its head; it will take it anyhow! So the sufferer should go along with it willingly, until memory has done its worst and courage and understanding have reasserted themselves.

I am often asked why a nervously ill person can feel so well one day and yet so ill the next. As already mentioned, yesterday's success can make a patient more vulnerable to failure today. This is one of the paradoxes that makes recovery from nervous illness so difficult to understand. The reason is that the nervously ill person resensitises himself by being anxious to do as well today as yesterday. It is important to re-emphasise that the patient must practise and not test himself. If agoraphobic, he must not set an examination to see if he can travel without panic. If he has panic after panic while out, but practises taking panic the right way, as far as future recovery is concerned, the journey made with panic is just as successful as the journey made without it. When he tests himself, failure brings a sense of defeat, whereas failure with practice means only that he need practise again. The very thought of testing brings tension, the thought of practising holds no urgent demand.

A patient who says, 'I came in by train by myself today

and I didn't panic, and I haven't panicked for two weeks!
is still vulnerable to panic; he dislikes it so much, he has
counted the days since he last panicked. The patient who
says, 'I came by myself today in the train. I had three
awful panics, but I thought, "Come on, and do your
worst!"' is on a sounder road to recovery than the man
who is glad he has not panicked.

As mentioned earlier, the most alarming of the pitfalls
to recovery is the return of panic, months, even years, after
what the patient hoped was its final appearance. This not
only shocks, *it reminds*. It reminds its victim of so much he
believed he had forgotten. The fear he adds before he has
time to collect himself and remember what he should do
resensitises him and almost invariably he makes the old
mistake of capitulating before it and trying to run away
from it.

One woman, after being well for a year, had a return of
panic while shopping. She hurried from the shop and then
avoided that shop for months. She had run from fear in
fear. This mistake is easily made and is so damaging to
recovery. The reappearance of panic (natural enough in
itself) is perhaps the main reason for so many therapists'
pessimism in curing agoraphobia. Dr Marks[1] wrote, 'Agoraphobics do not respond particularly well to desensitisation since they have a strong tendency to relapse
repeatedly. Prognosis is poorer where patients have multiple attacks of panic . . .' and again, 'Patients who had
recently overcome their fears sometimes reported that a
single panic attack might undo the effects of weeks of
treatment . . .'

I regard returns of panic as an almost inevitable part of
recovery and encourage the patient to see them this way
and use them, even welcome them (difficult, but possible)
as opportunities to practise once more coping with panic

the right way. The patient should be warned that although an unexpected return of panic may shock and so, perhaps, resensitise him, he should never let it shock him so much that he withdraws from it in fear for long. He should understand that some tension, strain, has slightly sensitised his nerves once more, and that memory stirred by some sound, sight, smell, may have flashed panic almost reflexively. If panic comes like this to someone who has felt its overwhelming intensity in the past, he is apt to feel it just as intensely again when taken by surprise, because in him the way to panic is so well prepared. This is why I stress the necessity of learning how to cope with panic itself and not trying to get used to a feared situation. Recovery means being able to cope with panic and other nervous symptoms and does not necessarily mean their total abolition. How could it, when we must all feel stress and its symptoms while we live?

Another important cause of setback is the occurrence of flash-experiences which can also come when least expected. By flash-experiences I mean happenings difficult for the patient to describe: a sudden feeling of dissolution, of disaster, death, flashes of agitation, of unreality, obsession. These can come at any time, perhaps during an animated conversation when the patient may feel at his best and may have temporarily forgotten his illness. The effect can be so upsetting that he can be suddenly arrested in the middle of a sentence, a laugh, and may then think despairingly that he can go so far toward recovery, but will never completely recover. He should learn to see these strange moments as no more than flashbacks of no significance and to wait quietly for them to pass. If not allowed to baulk him unnecessarily, they will mean no more than the occasional unhappy, or strange, flash of memory most of us have from time to time. Many people have collected a few strange thoughts over the years which recur from habit and must be lived with. Treated as unimportant, they cause little disturbance.

It is a mistake to look for reasons for these flash-experiences; they should not be tracked down, analysed and so given unnecessary prominence. They are the result of the suffering the nervously ill person has been through and have no bearing on the future. The sufferer should be taught to pass through the moment of despair and go on quietly, without letting it spoil enjoyment. One woman wrote, 'Once in a while, I feel strange and I begin to panic and I think, "What do I do now?" When this happens I stay still because, if I don't, I'll push the wrong button and agitation and panic will follow. I'll be sitting at dinner with guests and suddenly I'll go silent. Something will have flashed into my mind that will have frightened me – one of my bogeys – and my husband will look and ask what's happened. I'll answer, "I just want to be quiet," and I wait until I realise what the next step is. It's usually something like, "You've been through this before! Don't hang on to it. Let it pass. There's nothing to it!" I know now what to do. I have the right tools and I'm using them at a slow pace and it's paying off!'

Sudden flashes of agitation may occur just as the patient is going off to sleep, or he may waken with one. Too often he will reach for a sleeping pill. Were he to wait as patiently as possible, the agitation would pass. It helps to discuss those moments with a patient.

Some of the symptoms of convalescence from a physical illness are the same as nervous symptoms; for example, palpitations, weakness, breathlessness, giddiness. A former nervous sufferer has only to feel these symptoms when convalescing from physical illness to be reminded of his nervous illness. Fear of the symptoms, together with possible debility brought by physical illness, may encourage a setback. It is wise, especially for a surgeon, to prepare such a patient for convalescence and explain that he need not feel overwhelmed at the thought of another long uphill climb back to health (having already made one uphill climb out of nervous illness), that nature will do the job if he is willing to step out of her way by not adding the stress of worrying about it.

It is essential for the nervously ill patient to appreciate the importance of habit, because so much of his illness is bound up in it. Fear of this, or that, is his habit. This is why he may seem to have things sorted out and see them clearly without fear for a while and then lose the glimpse. The habit of being afraid reasserts itself. When the patient appreciates the meaning of habit, he will understand why setbacks come and why progress seems to include so much going backwards into old habits. Habit dies hard, but it does die, if we see it through its violent protestations.

At school we are taught mathematics, history and so on, but rarely how to practise moderation. Moderation and self-discipline are the most important part of our defence mechanism. It is difficult not to be influenced by feeling. So many people are afraid of unpleasant feelings and suspect they may become more unpleasant if they face them, so they try to extinguish them before they become established. The mature person can free himself from emotional dictation and act after suitable deliberation.

If education included training in how to bear unpleasantness, and especially how *to let the first shock pass* until we could think more calmly, many an apparently unbearable situation would become manageable and many a nervous illness would be avoided, because nervous illness is, as I have tried to show in this book, so often no more than severe sensitisation perhaps accompanied by extreme mental fatigue, following prolonged, or sudden, possession by the stress of bewilderment and fear, specially fear of the sensitised state in which the sufferer finds himself.

The patient may think there is so much to remember, so much to do. There isn't. It is all in that one word *accept*. Once he has sufficient understanding, it will not matter if he forgets all other directions, as long as he remembers and practises acceptance.

CHAPTER TEN

Extract from lecture given at Queen Alexandra Hall, London, June 1973

This lecture was given to 100 agoraphobic men and women. I had treated them by remote direction for periods varying from a few months to seven years. They came from different parts of the United Kingdom Some had not travelled in a vehicle for years; others had not even left their homes to go down the street for years, before beginning treatment.

Ladies and Gentlemen:
When I tried to think about what I would say today, I thought, 'I don't suppose there will be one person coming who hasn't already read both my books, listened to my recordings. There is nothing new that I can say to these people and yet they will have come a long way!' Then I realised I had found the right approach. That was it! There is so much that is repetitive in this wretched illness and that alone bewilders, upsets and stops many people from recovering as quickly as they should.

If only you did have something different to cope with sometimes. It's repetition – the same pattern, same feelings, same places to try to go to, day after day. Even the repetition of failure, success, failure, success, becomes almost unbearable; the fact that some days you can cope, some days you can't. It's the same struggle, over and over.

Repetition of symptoms, the repetition of life in a village, suburb, town – coloured by the memory of the repetition of suffering – makes yours an illness of repetition. To help yourself recover, you must introduce enough success to break the cycle of drab repetition. The stumbling block for most nervously ill people, especially agoraphobics, is that they can't maintain success long enough to establish it as success. They have snatches of it, perhaps even months when they feel well. But then comes the setback and the same old repetition.

Unfortunately setbacks usually do come at some time or other. I know some people have stepped out of their illness like stepping out of an old pair of shoes. Complete understanding has cured them. But most of these are young people with much to live for and usually with stimulating work demanding their attention. What a help that is.

The average person has to go on with the same old daily chores; this way it's not easy to step out of illness quickly. No matter what you say to yourself before going to sleep, the old shoes are waiting in the morning, the old thoughts, old fears, old tasks. This is not easy. THIS IS NOT EASY.

But by quietly going on, quietly persisting, not being too discouraged by it (or as little as you can manage), you gradually pack in enough small successful experiences to begin to wipe out the dreaded repetition of failure. The new shoes are ready at last.

Look closely at this repetition. You will find that what upset you about your illness last year is probably upsetting you this year, and this takes a lot of understanding and a lot of courage because repetition is so tiring. Try doing one task over and over again and see how tired you become. To manage well in the bus last week and not so well this week is upsetting and therefore tiring, and once tired you are a sitting target for the return of symptoms. In other words, you have to let enough time pass until you can write up enough successes to more than balance the failures to be able to take a setback philosophically. This is why letting time pass is so important and why I want you to try not to be too discouraged however much you may fail sometimes, or even however much you may still always seem to fail.

Some of you have only just managed to get here – with the help of a husband, friend, or alone. I hope you aren't expecting me to give you some new magic wand. I hope you're not expecting too much from just seeing me. Some have written and said, 'If I could just see you, Doctor, I know I'd be better!' That wouldn't do at all. Seeing me will, I hope, give you fresh heart, but you have to come back to yourself for real help. *You still have to find within yourself what it takes to recover, because it is within yourself that you must look for courage in the future.* I try to help you to gradually build a foundation of knowledge, understanding and courage within yourself until finally nothing can shake you for long. You will notice that I did not say nothing could ever shake you again. The only way to be not shaken again is to be no longer alive.

There is a door out of this illness. Out of any maze there is usually one door. However, there are also many side passages that lead to dead-ends, so many wrong doors that lead only back to another passage. No wonder you become bewildered. Of course the right door, the one leading to freedom, is the least inviting. It's a bare-looking, dreary door, an impossible door. It doesn't even look as if it could open. You think, 'It couldn't be this! The door over there on the left is much more attractive. I'll try that first!'

The unattractive door leading to freedom has a stark notice that says, 'UTTER ACCEPTANCE'. Not a very

encouraging notice, is it? But, oh, to find that door
and open it! How difficult it is to open the door labelled
'UTTER ACCEPTANCE'. You see, it's been used so seldom,
the hinges are rusty. Besides, there's such an inviting path
on the right, leading to a most attractive door with a
handy seat for jelly-legs. This door is labelled, 'NOT
TODAY!' and there is a second door beside that one that
says, 'And I don't think I'll be able to manage it tomorrow, either!'

Then there is that special door, the one called '*What's
the use?*'. It opens at a touch, so often has it been used.
Unfortunately, some people have little incentive at home
to help them get well. It's hard for a person living alone, or
a person whose daily life is uninteresting, to find the incentive to get well. Going out is sometimes an effort for any of
us. Many must overcome an initial inertia. Agoraphobic
people must feel this very strongly because, not only do
they have the normal inertia, they have also the fear of
going out to cope with. That is a difficult door to avoid,
'*What's the use?*', and it is especially inviting because it
often leads to a nice cup of tea, fire and television. Never
take the door that says '*What's the use?*', go on, through the
next door. It says, 'MAKE THE EFFORT'.

Then there is the door that says, 'I have tried. I really
have tried, Doctor! I've done everything you said, all I
could possibly do, and I'm no better!' There's a very com-
fortable seat in front of that door and it's especially
tempting because people think they really have earned it.
They did their best! But they didn't. They didn't try the
right way nor long enough. They went through all the
other doors, but never found the one marked 'UTTER
ACCEPTANCE'. They thought they were accepting, but as
soon as they felt their feelings (the panic, weakness, giddiness and so on) reach a climax, they withdrew. They

almost accepted, but not at the final point. And, of course, it's just at that final point that the door unlocks. They – some of them – even had their hand on the handle and gave it a turn, but they didn't turn it completely round. *They took their hand off at the critical moment*!

Now, suppose you did pass through the door that says, 'UTTER ACCEPTANCE', and quite a number of you, judging from your survey forms, did. You accepted; you found out what it meant to feel successful. Some of you made this journey to London with moments of exhilaration. You have done things you have never done before, and you probably thought, 'This is it!' But that wretched door has a habit of having children, grandchildren, great grandchildren . . . lots of little doors, all along the way, and you have to keep passing through them. You may be so shocked by the fact that, having accepted on so many occasions, you meet further obstacles that seem to take just as much effort to accept that you think, 'Oh, no! Not again!' and your impulse is to turn aside. But all side passages lead back into the same maze and eventually back to the same door 'UTTER ACCEPTANCE'. So, beware of side passages. Whenever you are faced with a door marked 'ACCEPTANCE' go through. Take a deep breath, let your body go loose and float through.

I want to impress this on you today. Complete recovery means going through the door marked 'UTTER ACCEPT-ANCE' whenever it appears. And this brings me back to the beginning of this talk when I spoke about repetition.

You repeat acceptance and see its effect on your symptoms so often that you finally lose your fear of them, you see acceptance work so often you come to understand and believe in it. *Here, repetition is your friend*. Also, remember, stress must come from time to time, that's natural, and because the symptoms of stress are the symptoms of nervous illness when under severe stress you may think your illness has returned. Expect to feel the old symptoms when under stress. Never be shocked into thinking, 'Oh, my goodness! I'm going to have one of my old turns! Here it is again!' Try to remember that your turns are no more than the symptoms of stress and continue to accept them in the future as you are learning to accept them now.

I have just been talking about the future. Many of you are still worrying about coping with the present. You have accomplished wonders to come this far today and I congratulate you and appreciate the effort you have made. I know that to do this many of you had to practise much acceptance. When you return home don't forget this effort too quickly and lose heart again. Let today's effort help you face that door marked 'UTTER ACCEPTANCE' whenever you meet it; let it help you turn the handle right round and walk through. Remember, peace lies on the other side of that door.

CHAPTER ELEVEN

Extracts from 1970 Survey of 528 Agoraphobic Men and Women Treated by Remote Direction

These extracts give examples of the patients' estimation of their own progress, either satisfactory or good. Of the 528 men and women treated by remote direction, the results were satisfactory or good in 73% of those aged 17–28, 67% in those aged 30–39, 55% in those aged 40–49 and 49% in those aged 50–74. The majority of these people were chronic agoraphobics and presented a special challenge to treatment by remote direction.

Satisfactory Progress
Sex, female. Age, 60. Length of illness, 27 years. Time of treatment by remote direction, 4 years.

Previous treatment: 'A few months from a therapist who said he knew the kind of treatment I needed, but that he hadn't the time to treat me, because it was long term.'

What can you do now that you could not do before treatment by remote direction? 'I can do all my own shopping. Visit my general practitioner's surgery and hairdresser on my own. I can now do a long journey with a companion and enjoy staying away from home, either at my son's or my sister's, about 100 miles away.'

What is your attitude to setback? 'I accept it and wait for it to pass. I haven't felt panic since I started this method, but after all this time, four years, I still feel apprehension before starting on my own.'

Satisfactory Progress

Sex, female. Age, 25. Length of illness, 11 years. Time of treatment by remote direction, 6 years.

Previous treatment: 'Six psychiatrists. Eighteen months in a psychiatric hospital on drugs, E.C.T., group therapy, psychoanalysis, psychotherapy. The drugs and E.C.T., helped the depression, but nothing helped the phobias, especially agoraphobia.'

What can you do now that you could not do before treatment by remote direction? 'Go on holiday. Go to work; able to be alone sometimes. Get over depression much quicker. Mix with people without feeling different. I've had drugs for so long, I still rely too much on them.'

What is your attitude to setback? 'At first, I think, "Oh no! I'm going to be really ill again!" and then I remind myself that after a setback I nearly always feel better than before it.'

Satisfactory Progress

Sex, female. Age, 46. Length of illness, 19 years. Time of treatment by remote direction, 2 years.

Previous treatment: 'I have been in hospital for "nerves" and have been treated by several psychiatrists.'

What can you do now that you could not do before treatment by remote direction? 'My own shopping locally. Visit the hairdresser's. Went on a $3\frac{1}{2}$ hour train journey with my husband for the first time in 22 years. Going again at Easter.'

What is your attitude to setback? 'Try again.'

Good progress (Patient says, 'Cured, I hope.')

Sex, female. Age, 57. Length of illness, 40 years. Time of treatment by remote direction, 7 years.

Previous treatment: 'Not for agoraphobia.'

What can you do now that you could not do before treatment by remote direction? 'In my car, I can go anywhere. I really can't think of anything I could not tackle at the moment. I might still get a few twinges at the beginning, but once away I know I'll be O.K., so I just forget them. I doubt if my family ever knew I was as ill as I was.'

What is your attitude to setback? 'I treat it as normal. I don't worry about it. I know I'll be better the next minute, hour, or day!'

Good Progress

Sex, female. Age, 53. Length of illness, 12 years. Time of treatment by remote direction, 4 years.

Previous treatment: 'From a general practitioner for 12 years. This did not help me. From more than one psychiatrist for eight years, on and off, with hospitalisation. This did not help either.'

What can you do now that you could not do before treatment by remote direction? 'I can go on holiday without apprehension – even look forward to this year's holiday. I made a journey to England last year. I had been trying to do this for six years. I threw myself in at the deep end last year and just went, fear or no fear, relying on Dr Weekes's method and some tranquillisers.'

What is your attitude to setback? 'I can accept it now without losing my temper, or hope, and thinking, "If I don't make it today, I will tomorrow!"'

Good Progress

Sex, female. Age, 41. Length of illness, 15 years. Time of treatment by remote direction, 4 years.

Previous treatment: 'Psychiatrist for 12 years. Haven't been for two years. I was in hospital for seven months. It helped.'

What can you do now that you could not do before treatment by remote direction? 'Stay alone. Cope with panic flashes and setbacks. Go out more, think of others far more than I could before. Study music, cope with problems, support others, etc.'

What is your attitude to setback? 'I naturally don't like it, but I know I'll feel better given time, because I always do. I accept them on the advice I've had since doing it by Dr Weekes's method. My family and friends think I'm a different person.'

CHAPTER TWELVE

Scripts of Recordings used in Treatment by Remote Direction

(1) MOVING TOWARD FREEDOM

First, I must stress that I expect you to have been examined by your doctor, and told that you are suffering from nerves. I haven't the opportunity to examine you, so I must trust you to be examined by your own practitioner.

You have probably read my two books, played my records and have been trying to follow my advice, but you feel you need more ready help to move away from home, and keep moving once you are out, so here I am, ready to go with you.

If you are going out today, you have probably been thinking a lot about it and are already getting yourself worked up, because this may be a special occasion. It may be the first time you have this cassette to help you and you are probably wondering if it will really do its job. First, I want you to do this – don't try too hard now to alter your feelings before you set out, or even to pluck up courage. Be as worked up as you feel you must be, even despair when you feel like it. I know that one minute you think that you might make it, and the next you are sure that you won't. You think, 'What if the cassette doesn't help me! What will I do then?' You could hardly think any other way in the circumstances but, at the same time, under all those frightening thoughts, hold on to one special thought: 'I am going out today, however I feel. I'm really going. I'll make a start!' Good. I'm here beside you. We'll go together and we'll make it together.

Have you decided where we are going? Decide this before you set out. Ready? Now take it gently, don't go too quickly. Let go that tight grip, let it go! It doesn't matter how you feel at this moment, you won't always feel like this. You could hardly feel any other way now. So, come along with all those strange feelings. None of the feelings, horrible though they may be, can hurt you.

It's not easy for me to imagine where you are now. However, I'm going to suppose that you are walking down the street alone.

Don't be afraid to open your eyes and look about you. Stand up straight, let your arms drop loosely. Up, straight, that's it. Don't mind if the cars swish past; you'll get used to those gradually. After a few days, you'll take those for granted. Don't be frightened if you feel bewildered, even unsteady, *none of it matters*. Fear and tension have made you this way and your reactions now are normal reactions in the circumstances and don't think you're so very sick because you have these particular sensations. I want you to gradually release all that tension and find new wings.

From the moment you make up your mind to loosen to the best of your ability, your body will begin to recover. That's a good thought, isn't it? You really begin to recover the moment you release the tension and you do that by going quietly, slowly, being prepared *to let all feelings come*. Your feelings have been your master. They've been bluffing you, and yet you have been creating them yourself. The more tensely you withdraw from them, the more acute you make them. The way you create tension when you withdraw is rather like squeezing a lemon. I could put it this way: tension squeezes the glands that produce the chemicals that make the feeling of panic. So the more you work yourself up, the harder the squeeze, and the more panic, giddiness, weakness and so on. So, take your hand off that squeezer. Loosen, loosen – that's the way to do it. It doesn't matter if you fail as long as you try again the right way. When I tell you to go slowly, quietly, I'm really telling you to take time to think about panic, not run away from it. So, let your tummy feel loose, let it sag, feel as if it's sinking. Take in a deep breath and, as you breathe out, let go. Do this when you feel the panic mounting, when you feel it flash. Is it so difficult? Then if it is, try again. Go forward, almost as if you are floating forward. I don't expect you to do it this way all the time. I mean in those moments of great fear. You may have times when you feel yourself walking normally.

Suppose we go into a shop. Is there one near? Now, don't panic when you think of this. YOU CAN DO IT. The same magic will always work. Pluck up your courage now, but loosen, and quietly float in. YOU CAN DO IT. If you wait for a moment, take a few deep breaths. Expect to feel strange. You must feel strange, if you haven't been in a shop on your own for a long time! And remember, this is a practice, not a test!

Don't pity yourself and think, 'Why can't I be like all those other people! Why do I have to go through all this! Why do I have to carry a cassette!' If we don't get one thing in life, we get another! The big thing is to accept what has happened and now to come up out of it. NEVER RUN HOME IN FEAR; see it through and you will know what it's like to be really free. But freedom must be earned and the permanent way is the hard way. It has to be hard, because you have to find strength and strength is built on trying and tackling the hard things and this takes time.

Strength grows. It can't come out of the air. It must first come from your deciding to practise the right way, and then from your trying to do it.

Suppose we go a little further? Don't be surprised if the panic-blasters don't come. You may understand so well that you may find that you lose your fear of them. This could happen. You could be quickly cured. I have seen this happen. But if the old blasters do come, remember – they will always pass IF YOU WAIT. The trembling won't hurt you. Sit down if you feel you must, even have a sweet or two and then on, again. Here is hope. This way lies freedom.

Even when you successfully pass through the barrier, don't be upset if you meet it again while we're out. You know the barrier I mean – that feeling of being rigidly set in concrete, as if you can neither go forward nor backward, of being almost swallowed up by fear. Even when you manage this moment, don't be upset if it comes again and again on this journey. This is one of the strange things about recovery; you seem to have to go over and over the same experience and for a while it may seem just as difficult each time. I promise you that eventually it won't be hard. It takes time to reach this stage, so you must practise and practise. One of these days, when you do it the right way, you'll think, 'That's it! That's the way! I did it!' and once you've felt this, you'll want to be up and at it again. In time, you will have come through that barrier so often that you will automatically know the way through, and the only way is to go quietly up to it, accepting panic and all the other feelings as I'm trying to teach you.

So, when you panic, take a deep breath, let your body go loose, wait, and then go on. It's like playing golf – you know how to swing a club, but to do it the right way every time is a different matter. It takes practice. Sometimes you have the trick of going forward the right way for weeks and think you are really out of the wood, and then for some unaccountable reason you have another flash of panic. If this happens, try not to be shocked. Once again, WAIT, and practise going slowly again. Don't run away in fear! If you don't run away, although the panic may return from time to time, it won't shock you into being so afraid of it. It's an old bogey, really, because your fear of it creates it.

So, be reconciled to taking the hard road today and tomorrow, until the day comes when you feel it isn't hard any more. Let your body go loose, take a deep breath, let it out – there, it wasn't so bad was it? I promise you, it isn't so difficult when you learn to do it the right way. When you learn how to cope with panic and all the other sensations that you dread, you gradually do lose your fear of them, and when you are unafraid there is no longer any IT, because IT is the fear you create.

You've been like a puppy chasing its tail, round and round, chasing the fear – the fear you make, because you are afraid of the feelings of fear. Courage, old soldier! Don't be downhearted when you fail. You belong to a very special group. So many march beside you today, doing it this way, so don't feel too lonely.

If I were actually with you, I couldn't give you more encouragement than I want to give you now. You have it all. YOU CAN DO IT. Nobody need fail, however big a coward he may think himself.

(2)   GOING ON HOLIDAY

Now, I'll talk about going on holiday. Let's suppose that you've told the family that you'll go and you're faced with those weeks before leaving – the big build-up to going.

You will eventually be able to take holidays with the family, or by yourself, but before you can do this you must begin by learning how to go through that strange period before the holiday of 'Will I? Won't I? Can I? Can't I?' – a spasm of hope one minute, a glimpse that you could make it and, the next minute, that leaden feeling of certainty that you won't. Shilly-shally if you must. At this moment you may not be able to do it any other way. That last week, those last few days, won't be easy, so don't expect them to be. And because they are so hard, don't think that you are particularly ill or that holidays are never for you. Considering the way you've suffered in the past, how could you approach a holiday any other way than this? But underneath, hold on to that little seed of determination, that however you feel, whatever you think, this time, you are going. Sometimes you may think, 'Well, they'll have to carry me there!' All right! But if you decide that, carry or no carry, you're really going, I promise that when the day eventually comes you may go off in a sort of dream, but you will go, and it won't be half as bad once you get started as it is waiting for time beforehand to pass. So please, please, just quietly go through the hours, days, through shilly-shally, but underneath trust what I teach you and make up your mind to go. Be two people. One that suffers and, underneath the suffering, the one that is going. If you do this you'll be surprised at the way you'll be able to take the holiday and get benefit from it. At the moment you may be feeling desperate at the thought of going. Let the moments of desperation pass. Don't clutch them and they will pass.

Have you seen your doctor about tranquillisers to help you during these few weeks? You may need a sleeping pill the night before you go. I hope your doctor understands. If he knows what you are trying to do, he should help you. So, pass through the desperate moments, and let the person under all that shilly-shally take over. There is a person there capable of taking over, even though you may doubt it. Quietly, let that person come up. You only need a tiny grain of resolution to get you there if you go the way I teach you.

When the morning comes at last, you may either think, 'I've come so far! Here goes for the rest!' and you may be off with quite a dash. Or, you may set off as if it's all happening to someone else. Go in a dream, if it's like that, *but go*. If you turn back in failure, you'll be so upset with yourself, so desperate, you'll hardly know what to do, or where to go to hide from yourself or the family. Going away is less of an ordeal than going through the purgatory of failing to go, so avoid that pit of despair whatever happens! Say to the family, 'Whatever I do, whatever I say, make me go!'

The feeling of almost paralysis that may come when you think about moving, or when the actual morning arrives and you try to go, is no more than supertension and you've built it up yourself. This is where I want you to remember the word 'float'. Let your body go, loosen that tight hold. Now move forward in a floating kind of way. This is the way to undo the tension when you feel bound up in it. It's the tension that makes you feel as if some outside force is holding you back. That's all it is. Strange, isn't it? To think you build this up within yourself, the thing you least want, the chains that bind, you create yourself from fear of them. So don't draw back. It doesn't matter how you feel at this moment. Go! You'll be so glad when you do.

There will be so much to do around the place in those weeks before leaving. Take it a moment at a time. Slowly. It doesn't matter how slowly. Pack the suitcase, a moment at a time. If you can't think, wait till you can. A cup of tea helps you to pass through one of those concrete moments; you know the moment – when you think you'll never move freely again. But even that moment melts if you take it slowly. Wait! Go limp and breathe deeply. You'll know that off by heart, won't you? I hope you do. This is the way to get better. On, always on, through it all but not with clenched teeth! With looseness and willingness to try to accept.

A man wrote recently and said, 'I didn't believe it could be so simple! I feel that I've been let out of prison!' It is simple, if you do it this way. You notice that man said 'simple'. He didn't say 'easy'. It's simple but *it's not easy*. Another woman said, 'I remember what Dr Weekes says until I panic. Then I can't remember a word!' But I only want you to remember two words, just two words – *loosen, accept*. You have only to remember those. It doesn't matter if you think you can't loosen, if you accept even that! You could leave your journals and your books, even this tape behind, if you remembered to take with you, engraved on your mind and heart, ACCEPT. Nothing would happen to you. Perhaps a few flashes might be as strong as ever, but they would die down sooner. You would have learnt the trick.

Did we make it? Are we on holiday now? Well, even if you are only listening to this cassette out of interest, I can tell you about being on holiday, and if you listen often enough, by the time the next holiday comes around, you may be ready to go. Do you remember the woman in the journal who couldn't make the town centre? She flew to Spain a few weeks ago, so you see, this method does work.

Let's suppose you have gone on holiday. One part of you will feel happy to think you did, and the other part may be afraid for fear you now spoil it all by having to run back home. Don't turn back! Keep your case packed if you feel safer that way. But WAIT. In a little while you'll feel less strange. In a few days it won't all seem so far from home. It is surprising how a place that seems cold and unfriendly can change after you've been in it for a few days. You begin to know the girl at the reception desk, your room doesn't seem so strange, even the shops begin to look familiar. And the knowledge that you *have* stayed begins to seep through and agitation begins to settle. You count the days to going home and, as each day passes, the number of days grows less and then you begin to think, 'Well, I may as well see it out!' and, wonder of wonders, you may even begin to enjoy it. It gradually seems more homely. It's those first few days that are the worst. After that, the place becomes a place you know.

Pass through those first few days. If you find this time very hard, at least you are listening to this tape. This should comfort and help you. Now, I'm going to let you into a secret. You are going to stay, so you may as well accept it all! You guessed I wouldn't let you go home, didn't you? So, wait a little longer, and on with the things that have to be done. Try not to be too impressed with the way you feel. Just for a little while longer. *They are only feelings* and feelings can change.

You may find that you can enter these shops more easily than you can enter the shops near home. You may think this extraordinary, but it isn't extraordinary. Memory isn't hiding in these shops to try to drag you back. You won't bump into an inquisitive neighbour here. This is a freedom you haven't had for a long time! It's a taste of something to get better for, isn't it? Stay! And in a little while you may find the courage to go on a short bus ride. Impossible? Not at all! You can do it, if you remember those two words – loosen, accept. You may even have tea in a crowded tea shop, near the door of course – I'll allow you that much, this time! Hot scones, strawberry jam. It will seem strange doing this. But after a while you may think, 'If only I could stay like this for ever! Do I have to go back home?' It is a pity holidays are so short. It's not easy to go back into the trap that you think is waiting. But if you return the right way, it won't be quite the same old trap. In the meantime we won't worry about going home. You may still have those first few days to get through without turning back.

If you do have panic-blasters while you're away, don't immediately think you have failed. Let the old panics come, let them come. Never be disappointed by a flash of panic. I'd like to embroider that in gold and give it to you to wear as a bracelet, because recovery means learning how to cope with blasters. Never think a blaster means failure and that the end of the world has come. It's good practice taking the unexpected panics. So go on once more. The person who recovers is the one who goes on, on, on, practises again and again.

Now, when you go home, don't lose the holiday spirit too quickly. Do something a bit daring every few days. I don't know what you'll find daring to do – but try. Don't slip back into the old routine too soon and don't let the old familiar places upset you too much, your old failure places, the shop where you panicked, the crossing where you usually panic. Of course you failed there, you panicked there, but when you are afraid once more in these places try to remember that this is memory up to its tricks again. If you panic on returning home, come through it the same old way I've been teaching you, have always been teaching you. You remember? The two words, loosen and accept.

Well, we've been down the street and we've been on holiday – perhaps! But if you do no more than listen to this tape often enough, you may be ready to take a holiday sometime in the future. Good luck.

(3)   GOOD NIGHT, GOOD MORNING
       (for those afraid of the state they are in)
Short talk

Good morning. This first talk is a short one, just to help you get out of bed and to be with you while you are dressing. It will be followed by a longer talk to play during the morning – if you have the opportunity – or maybe while you're having breakfast you may choose to play special sections from it. This first short talk is to help you out of bed.

Another day is here, so what are you going to be afraid of today? If you examine what frightened you yesterday, was it so terrible? If you examine it honestly, you'll find that it was no more than fear added to fear. Let's face it. That's what it was. Your symptoms are the symptoms of fear and your fear of them keeps them going. That's it, in a nutshell!

After all, what you went through yesterday didn't kill you, did it? *Don't let fear bluff you.*

The key is still in those words, loosen and accept. Take a deep breath . . . let it out slowly . . . and as you let it out, let your tummy muscles sag, loosen, let your arms go *loose at the shoulders*. This is the feeling I am talking about when I mention 'floating'. Now, I want you to go through *any* fears you might have today *in this way*. In this way, go through any frightening suggestions you may make to yourself, such as 'Oh no! Not another day! How am I going to cope with it?' Take a deep breath, let it out slowly, let your tummy muscles go loose and that's how you're going to cope with it. Any surfer knows that he doesn't fight the big waves; he goes under them. Go under, or float past your fear; don't fight. A deep breath, let it out, let your shoulders sag, and let it all come, let the wave go over and past.

Today I want you to do something special. I want you to

go right through the peak of experience – by that I mean the climax to any fear – in just that way. Take a deep breath, let it out slowly and take today and its fears with utter, utter acceptance.

Today is one more bead to push along the string, letting time pass. If your body is so tired that you feel you can't get out of bed, be cheered, this is only nervous tiredness. (Once more I assume you have been examined by your doctor.) You can get yourself up. You did it yesterday and all the other yesterdays . . . so, a deep breath and up!

Remember, you have only fear of the symptoms of fear to fear. Don't be bluffed by fear.

Longer talk

Once more, good morning! This isn't going to be the kind of talk that says 'Isn't it wonderful to be alive?' There *is* joy in living; there is joy in so many things and it's there for you too. But, first, you may have to get through a period of thinking that there's not much joy anywhere. All you may want to do now is to be able to get up with the courage to face the day.

First, I want to make it clear that I am taking for granted that you have been examined by your doctor and that he has told you that your trouble is nervous; that physically you are sound. A person suffering from nerves must be sure that he, or she, does not suffer from some organic illness, something that can be treated medically and so speed recovery.

It's true that nervous depletion alone can make you feel exhausted – so tired you may think you can hardly drag your body off the bed – and it's difficult to believe that such great tiredness can be caused by nerves. If you are as exhausted as this, you probably think that there must be something physically wrong with you.

However, nervous tiredness can make even a young, healthy person feel as tired as if he were 90 years old. So, if you have confidence in your doctor and he has definitely assured you that yours is nervous exhaustion, then however tired you may be understand that nerves really can make you feel this way, and that it doesn't harm you to work through the day. But here again, moderation in all things . . . and I advise you to take short rests when you feel most tired if, of course, this is practicable.

And when you get up and start to move round, if you feel you can move about only slowly, then move slowly, but *willingly*. By degrees, as the morning passes, your metabolic rate – that's the rate at which your cells produce energy – will speed up and you won't feel quite so helpless, so powerless. Sometimes, by night, some nervous people's metabolic rate has so far recovered and they feel so much better that they want to prolong the evening; indeed, they dread going to sleep because they know that when they do the morning will come all too soon and they will once more feel tired, perhaps even depressed.

If you feel your worst in the morning, don't judge yourself by how you find yourself at this stage in your illness. Try not to worry about how you feel. You'll notice how you feel, of course you will, who wouldn't? But when you do notice, try not to be too depressed about it, or too discouraged by it.

Maybe you are lonely, lack confidence, perhaps you're even without much hope of getting through the day successfully. But I hope you are prepared to try to accept the way you feel now; that you are willing to try to get through this day to the best of your ability. This is the way to get through the day at this stage; simply work to the best of your ability, BUT WILLINGLY.

If you are a housewife you may be facing a day that doesn't hold much interest, perhaps not even enough interest to make you do your hair properly. Your body will heal itself even of apathy and lack of interest, *if* you will let it. *All the time* your body is trying to heal itself, to give you a new spirit, fresh heart. And it can do it, if you will let it. So, get up, dress, make a cup of tea, or coffee if you prefer, and try to point the body willingly. However, you don't have to put on an act! You don't have to try to *force* hope. When you try to force hope, you will succeed only in being hopeful one minute and despairing the next. Having spurts of hope and despair doesn't help one little bit. If you are truly hopeful – if you feel hope deep within you – that's different. It's good. But don't think you must try to be hopeful. Getting better means taking whatever comes, hope or despair. You can't force hope because hope won't stay if you do.

Hope is a very evanescent feeling to the nervously ill person. It's here at three o'clock and gone at a minute past three. You don't need that kind of fleeting hope to help you recover. So, don't despair if hope goes quickly. However, in time, when you work the way I teach you, hope stops fleeting and becomes an inner feeling of strength. But it takes time for this feeling to become established. In the meantime, you begin to recover *on deep understanding* and you start to get this understanding by deciding that you *are* going to try to do it today the way I have been teaching you.

I'm not saying, 'Wake up, the sun is shining! On, with a positive feeling of joy in this and joy in that!' That wouldn't last two minutes. I'm saying, 'This day for you might not be so good. There may not be much energy, much interest, much strength, but try to understand that, at this stage, the day probably couldn't be much different from this.' However, you can attack the day differently. If you practise doing what I tell you now, in time the mornings will be very different.

So, go quietly through the day, accepting all, and when you do it this way, an unknown power within you will be doing the work of healing. *You* don't have to do the actual healing yourself. You wouldn't know how to. You haven't got quite the uphill job you think you have, have you? Your body will heal itself, if you step out of its way . . . and you step out of its way by *accepting that poor old body as it is today*.

While you try to accept, be cheered by the knowledge that you're accepting a miracle worker that will move mountains for you, if you give it the chance . . . and you give it this chance by practising utter, utter acceptance. Today, simply work to the best of your ability this way. If you're working at home, sit down when you feel you must, even lie down when you feel you must; don't force yourself to work with gritted teeth – but don't lie or sit for too long.

Even while you rest, if you rest *willingly*, and don't worry because you are resting, you are still on the march forward. You must be, because those unseen forces work all the time as long as you play them the WILLINGLY TUNE. They will go on healing, as long as you don't add too much despair and throw them out of gear. Fear, despair, frustration – those are the spanners that get thrown into the works and, of these, the worst is fear.

But remember that you cope with fear by accepting it whenever it comes. I have explained this in my books and records so often. We all carry fear with us, but the nervously ill person adds *second-fear*; he is afraid of fear, afraid of the sensations fear brings. *Don't be bluffed by fear*. Panic is a superficial feeling. Even though it may seem overwhelming, consuming and very deep-seated indeed, it is no more than a superficial electrical discharge felt mainly at nerve endings . . . *it is only skin deep*! So, panic is simply an electrical discharge and, as such, has a limited strength even though you may not think so; so why let an electrical discharge, a mechanical thing, spoil your life, when by loosening and accepting it you actually take your finger off the controlling switch.

Here is a letter from a woman who finally made a journey abroad. She said, 'I was having a wonderful time, but suddenly one night, as I entered the dining room, I had a terrible feeling of self-consciousness – and it was my favourite dinner – roast turkey! I just couldn't swallow it, so I did the only thing I could think of, I ate the soft vegetables and the dessert and kept repeating 'Loosen and accept, loosen and accept!' and by the time we'd had coffee, I was fine! I had a fantastic holiday.'

You see, she could have failed at that moment, but she loosened and accepted fear; and that is what I'm asking you to do today.

Of course, if you have felt panic for a long time, it may still give you a good old blaster now and then for some time to come, but with your hand off the switch, that is, with acceptance in your heart, the strength of the current will gradually die down.

It may take time for panic to cease coming altogether, but as time passes, panic upsets you less and less when you *know* that *you* know how to cope with it. You loosen and accept.

Now, you *are* going to give it that chance today, aren't you? Time and acceptance are the answers. So don't judge yourself as you find yourself this morning. Oh no! Give more time! When you went to bed last night, I asked you only to hope for the courage to accept yourself as you would find yourself this morning didn't I? So, please try to do *just that*.

This is another day, another bead along the string. Do what you have to do to the best of your ability. If you have to get the children to school, or get yourself off to work, plod along and do it. It won't always be a plod.

Ordinary life is not very interesting when one is depleted. Ordinary life may never be very interesting for some of us but, if we do things for people we love, it is not quite such a burden. However, if you're doing things for people you don't love, life can indeed be difficult. And if you feel this way, do something about it, but not until you are well enough to make sensible plans. It is difficult to make big changes, big decisions when nervously ill, and it is therefore wisest not to make them now, unless they are definitely impeding recovery.

And today, don't be too fussy about your work. At this stage don't set too high a standard for yourself; don't demand too much in the way of performance at work. What's more, you don't have to be especially cheerful about it. As long as you do it *willingly*, the rest will gradually follow. And if loneliness is part of your trouble, don't have the mistaken idea that living alone can send you mental. It can't. I mention this because so many lonely people have written asking this question. Some people even think that talking to themselves is the first sign. Well, I talk to myself quite frequently, if that's any comfort to you. None of these things matters; it hardly matters what you do, as long as you don't worry because you do it! It's the worry that tires, sensitises. And even if you are lonely and think you are trying to recover alone – you aren't. Hundreds are playing this record possibly at this minute and they will be trying to follow my teaching with you. So take heart; you have their company.

Suppose you are going out to work today. I don't know

what work you do, whether it's interesting or not. But I do know that if you tackle your work without worrying about whether it is interesting, the time will come when you will have the courage, motivation and the ability to find work that you like, because you will be more poised, more confident within yourself for having coped with yourself at a time when it was most difficult to cope, and that, of course, is *now*.

And if there are people at work who upset you, or whom you may fear, cope with them by practising floating past your reactions to them. By this I mean try to be detached from your feelings about them. When most upset, take a deep breath, let it out slowly, let your body go loose, and *let the shudder pass*. Don't be too impressed by how you feel when you contact these people. I know this is difficult to do, but you are especially helped if you have before you the goal of being able to do good work, however you may feel. It's the goal that matters, not the people, and *the goal is yours*. Don't let anyone rob you of that by letting them get under your skin too much. They're not worth it, but the goal is.

As a beginning toward reaching this goal, when you speak, speak up; don't hang your head and mumble. Get the habit of straightening up and looking people in the face. Look up, speak up. Yes. You can do it. In nervous illness one tends to be too hangdog, too low voiced; you think you haven't the confidence to speak up. Forget about confidence, don't wait for that to come. We can all find confidence, even you, if we want it enough. Lift up your head and speak out and confidence will follow. You have the power to do this, I know you have it. I've watched too many extremely self-conscious patients gradually learn how to straighten up and speak out. So, today, go to work charged with the inspiration to act, as I've just taught you. But don't go about it in an aggressive way. Don't force yourself tensely. I want you first to try to unscrew the screws, loosen the body and accept. Accept your shyness, accept your lack of confidence; don't fight them. Stand up and speak up WITH THEM THERE, HOWEVER YOU FEEL, STAND UP AND SPEAK UP. And when you do, you'll be surprised at the confidence that eventually develops within you.

So now at this moment, whether you are man or woman, work outside or inside the home, whatever you do, lift up your head, take a deep breath, let it out slowly, loosen your body and start this day willingly with acceptance to the very best of your ability. Take fear with you if you must, but don't let fear bluff you today. Let any nervous sensation come. Let it come. But pass through it, through . . . through. Loosen and accept. UTTER, UTTER ACCEPTANCE.

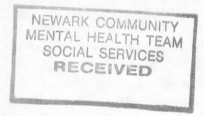

CHAPTER THIRTEEN

Digest of Journals (1972–74)
Used in Treatment by Remote Direction

During 1969–74 I sent quarterly journals to approximately two thousand nervously ill people in the British Isles, Ireland, America, Australia, New Zealand, Canada and South Africa. The original eight journals (1969–71) are printed in my second book *Peace from Nervous Suffering*. The following digest covers the remaining journals distributed during 1972–74. In this I discuss some specific problems common to many agoraphobic people.

The upstairs classroom

A schoolgirl of fourteen wrote, 'My main worries are at school. Would you please help me to stay in the upstairs classroom, Doctor?'

She said that using the method I had taught her she can now 'go to school to some lessons, go into town shopping, go for walks, cycle, go to movies, have visits from friends and visit friends.' Her attitude to setback is, 'I get cross but I look at it as only temporary.' That's good progress for a girl of fourteen.

I will now talk directly to her (and possibly to some of you in a comparable situation). You are on the way to complete recovery, but it is true that you must first cope with that upstairs classroom. Obviously upstairs worries you because retreat is difficult. Also, when you are out shopping, visiting, doing some of the new things you can now do, there is diversion and elation at 'doing' to help you. In the classroom upstairs there is only quietness, heads bent over books, and the teacher walking up and down the aisle, sometimes unexpectedly looking over your shoulder and asking questions. Everything is still and those wretched stairs are between you and freedom. So much time to sit and feel afraid! Upstairs is quite a place, isn't it?

The key to staying in the upstairs classroom is to take every worrying thought, every frightening feeling, *slowly*. At the first flashing signal (and this may come as you begin to mount the stairs, before you see upstairs) don't rush headlong into further panic and confusion. *Stay still! Wait!* Let that moment pass. Your reaction is now one of blind fear. You won't be able to stop fear coming for some time yet, but you can stop it from being *blind* fear. It's when you close your mind and wilt before the onslaught of fear, that you want to run away. *Stay with the fear.* Can you understand that? I mean have the courage to watch the fear. Then it will slowly pass. Fear doesn't like being watched. It's at its best when you shrink from it blindly: then it can put on its most terrifying act.

Once you are determined to stay upstairs and work quietly *with the fear there* – however, *accepting* the fear, not *fighting* it – you will be surprised how the panic will gradually settle into being an inner, boring, perhaps burning, churning kind of feeling which will be more easily borne than panic and which will in time quieten completely.

I don't mean that having faced and accepted panic in this way that the battle will be over and that you won't panic again. Of course, you may; perhaps many times during the same lesson. Accept each return of panic and go through it the same way. Remember, flashing panic can't kill you, can't hurt you, shows very little, if at all, on your face. Sometimes panic and other nervous symptoms make following a lesson difficult and the teacher may misjudge you and think you are wilfully not paying attention. You can't expect her to have second-sight, can you?

Be encouraged by knowing that you are doing magnificently simply by coming through a situation like this. This is the most important job you could do at the moment; it is even more important than learning your lessons. If you succeed only some times, you will have made great progress. It takes only a few successes to show you the way but usually much success to consolidate progress. So, never lose heart completely and finally you will be more mistress of yourself than most of the other girls in your class who have not had the opportunity to come through an experience like yours. It seems hard that one as young as you should have to suffer like this, but what you learn from it will be an insurance for the rest of your life, and what an understanding mother you will make.

So, go upstairs slowly (as slowly as the girls will allow as they scramble and push past) and let all the strange feelings come. Sit in your chair quietly, even if the frightening sensations seem to sizzle the roots of your hair. Go toward them. By that I mean relax your body as much as you can and don't shrink from the feelings. If you do this, you will find that by loosening yourself, letting your body feel as if it is sagging, the worst moments will calm and in time, upstairs will be no different from downstairs except, of course, for the memories it will hold. When that time comes, you must be ready to practise all I have told you about coping with memory and understand the tricks it will try to play.

So, young woman of fourteen years, don't avoid the

upstairs classroom. It is your special opportunity to practise coping with your nervous symptoms and finally becoming the true mistress of yourself. And remember,
when you are upstairs with all those girls hemming you in,
never give way to the urge to run, run, run. Instead, sit, sit,
sit. When you run, you are running away from yourself
not the upstairs classroom, and none of us has ever run far
from ourselves. Whatever you feel, remember *it is only a
feeling* brought on by your own fear of it. Have the courage
to accept it as willingly as you can manage. In this way
you gradually desensitise yourself and the feelings calm.
I have given you the tools. Now is the time to use them.

*'I can manage singing two verses of a hymn, but singing eight is too
much!'*

This woman has probably sung the first two verses man-
fully, standing tensely on guard, perhaps feeling giddy because of tension, and with every word a struggle. Small
wonder, with her imagination also at work, her mind
boggles at the thought of standing like this through
another six verses.

A walking tour, however long, can be made only a step
at a time. Eight verses can be sung only a word, a phrase,
at a time. She should not concentrate on the remaining six
verses ahead but on each phrase as she sings it. If tension
mounts, she should take a deep breath, let it out slowly, let
her body sag, and practise floating past the thought of the
perils her imagination is conjuring up. Slowly, slowly, a
deep breath, a sagging body, a phrase at a time and understanding that she creates the tension that defeats her with
her own apprehension.

Examination by your doctor
Some symptoms caused by nerves can also have organic

origin, so be sure to be examined by your doctor before you diagnose 'nerves'. For example, giddiness can be caused by wax on an ear drum, blocked eustachian tube, tensed neck muscles, low blood pressure; eyesight may need checking, old glasses corrected, and so on. Tension from anxiety can itself cause giddiness, so much that it may seem difficult to turn without swaying. Be sure to be examined by your doctor.

Going out alone without giving it a thought
'I wonder how long it will be before I can go out alone like other people, without giving it a thought?' Going out alone without giving it a thought means being so far removed from suffering (so much time having passed in recovery) that an agoraphobic has almost forgotten being afraid to travel by himself.

For a long time yet, this woman will go out remembering and watching herself. Recovery does not mean quickly forgetting being unable to go out alone. Recovery means first passing through several stages. In the beginning footsteps falter and from this woman's letter I'd judge her to be at this stage. Then come days of success mixed with days of failure and then, such success that the adventurer thinks incredulously, 'Is this me, doing this alone!' That's a good feeling; however, it's only after much repetition of such success that the once-agoraphobic person reaches the final stage of being able to take going alone for granted. First, she must go through those early stages.

Strangely enough, when an agoraphobic reaches the stage of automatic doing, he, or she, may complain about losing the earlier feeling of elation, may even say they feel 'flat'. However, for some of you, there will always be that thrill when you stop to think of how little you could once do and how much you can do now. This is your compensation. The fear and awareness of travelling alone changes into joy at awareness of doing it alone.

One woman said, 'I went to my son's prize-giving and watched him get a prize. For two hours I sat hemmed in by people and I didn't panic once. I couldn't have done that a year ago. It was worth everything, when my son looked up at me later and said, "Gee, Mum! You're doing great!"'

So, take heart and don't envy your nonchalant fellow travellers. Can you let the knowledge that so many have 'made it' encourage you? Indeed, many have said they won't be needing journals this year, because they are cured.

My legs lock

'I'm afraid my legs will lock and I'll stay paralysed when I have to do something important!' Legs 'locked' by nerves are merely stiffened by tension (fear) and are never truly paralysed. If a mouse were to run across that woman's toes in one of her locked moments, she would soon find the use of her legs. No amount of tension can truly paralyse a limb. It can only bluff the sufferer into thinking it has.

However, this woman needs more help than the presence of a mouse. She needs to know what to do if her legs should 'lock', or feel they are about to lock. (She does not say that her legs have actually locked.)

I remind her of the word 'float'. Perhaps you remember the woman in my first book, *Self Help for Your Nerves*, who, when I asked her to buy some fish replied, 'I couldn't go into a shop! I haven't been inside one for years! My legs would go paralysed before I could get there!' I explained that if her legs stiffened at the entrance of the shop, she should take a deep breath, let it out slowly (the same old process), stretch her arms out a little and imagine she was floating in. She returned with the fish, saying, 'Send me for something else, quickly! While I'm still floating!'

Suppose the woman who wrote the letter about fear of her legs locking were to reply to my instructions, 'But I can't float! What will happen if my legs really do lock?' I assure her they would not stay locked for long. Excess tension soon fatigues tensely contracted muscles and her legs would relax automatically in spite of her fear. What a bogeyman she has let frighten her.

Thoughts strengthen

A man complained that when he tried to talk himself out of a setback his thoughts always seemed so weak. He asked, 'How can I strengthen my thoughts?' When we talk about thoughts strengthening we mean that our emotional response to thoughts calms so that thoughts, unhampered by emotion, come through more clearly and so seem stronger and can more easily direct us.

When first in a setback, you may say to yourself, 'I'm not going to let this get me down! I'm not going to feel depressed about it!' However, if you are sensitised and your emotions therefore too easily aroused, too intense, they can so easily swing down into acute despair and disappointment despite your best effort. And while despair is so easily aroused, successfully talking yourself out of it is a formidable task. You may succeed at three o'clock, only to fail at five minutes past three. This is why you should try not to be so impressed by your emotions *of the moment* and not doggedly persevere with self-argument while it seems persistently ineffective. Do you remember the woman who said that when setback struck, she went round all day giving herself words, words, words trying to lift herself out of it and getting nowhere? How much easier for her if she had not made that effort and had accepted her reactions at the time and concentrated on quietly letting as much time pass as setback demanded. In time when her emotions had calmed, encouraging thoughts would have seemed stronger and would have directed and supported her more successfully.

I must warn you here. Some people make the mistake of expecting emotions to calm and thought to seem stronger as soon as they begin to practise being less impressed by their feelings of the moment. They expect a miracle while they watch and wait for it. Emotions do not calm as quickly as this, even with utter acceptance a few weeks (perhaps longer) may have to pass before the sufferer feels appreciably calmer. If you are just beginning to practise being unimpressed by your emotional reaction of the moment, don't be too discouraged if you don't get immediate results. If you willingly accept an inability to think yourself quickly out of setback, improvement will not be so far away. When I speak of willing acceptance, I mean *willing* and this means letting as much time pass as your desensitation demands.

'If only I could drive a hundred miles and not just twenty!'
Few non-nervously ill people like driving a hundred miles alone. Only someone strongly motivated by necessity, or an ambitious agoraphobic with some success to his credit would want to. If I had to drive a hundred miles, I'd first see if a friend were going my way. That's not agoraphobia.

Were this woman needed urgently a hundred miles away, she'd make the journey. It's amazing what a recovering agoraphobic can do when urgent action is demanded and there is little time for contemplation and apprehension. Also, so much of an agoraphobic's success lies in repeated practice, and few have repeated opportunity of driving a hundred miles, especially alone. If such a journey were necessary for this woman, I suggest that she divide the hundred miles into packages of twenty and drive each package separately. I assure her that if she has the courage to accept the challenge, she will find that the actual journey is different from the imagined one. There is diversion on the way, the feeling of achievement, even occasional elation to help her and dividing the journey into twenty mile packages breaks up the seemingly endless vista.

In the meantime, she should concentrate on practising nearer home and leave driving a hundred miles until opportunity knocks. She thinks she can't manage now because she's driving in her imagination and you all know what a stumbling block imagination can be. In imagination she cannot see herself beginning the journey, much less completing it. Don't let imagination bluff you into inactivity.

Coping with guilt
Be as compassionate toward yourself as you are toward others. This is not easy. It helps to remember that what ever you did at a particular age, you did because you had developed only as far as that age. Growing up is learning to act guided by previous experience – or, it should be. One of life's ironies is that we learn more from our mistakes, failures, than from our successes. The effect of a mistake bites more deeply. I keep repeating that you learn as much, if not more, from setback as from success.

As for guilt, if you sometimes wonder how you could have acted as you did, then guilt has served its purpose; you have learnt from experience. Try not to let the thought of guilt of the past destroy the present, especially if the present affects other people. The present can be so much more constructive because of lessons learnt from past mistakes.

If you feel guilty because you think you could have treated someone now dead more kindly (as the writers of some letters have complained), be consoled. Many suffer that way. It's all too easy to forget the difficult tasks accomplished and remember only your short irritable replies, the snappy rejoinders. Nerves become sensitised by constant, small irritations; it's difficult to take constant irritations, although small, perhaps year after year. People are lucky who have no special duty that subjects them to such a trial. Men are usually luckier than women, because too often it's the daughter or sister – especially the unmarried woman – who fulfils the family obligations, particularly to elderly parents. It is the daughter's or sister's nerves that become sensitised. her patience sometimes at breaking point and her conscience later involved. She is so much more likely to remember what she failed to do, or did not do well, than the demanding work she accomplished. As I said earlier, she should try to be compassionate toward herself and remember that at least she took the burden.

Nervously ill people are especially susceptible to guilt. One woman said, 'For many years I have felt guilty because of my illness, a second class citizen, a poor fish, a weakling, etc. Although I'm much better, I can't rid myself of this guilt.'

The nervously disturbed are conditioned to think this way, because so many who have never been nervously ill regard nervous illness as a weakness, even as cowardice. How ironic this is. The bravery of many nervously ill people is phenomenal. Day after day, they may live with and try to fight nervous symptoms – electric panic, tensed muscles, sweating palms, pounding heart, churning stomach, throbbing head – and sometimes, through shame (especially if panic is present) or not wanting to upset the family — they don't even talk about it, or have given up talking about it to an unsympathetic audience. They struggle on alone, bewildered, despairing, but still ready to put their head on the block and try again if life demands it, especially if life with their family demands it. How ironic that they, of all people, should feel guilty.

I have always said that to suffer nervous illness is a privilege. I said this once to a young woman going through a particularly gruelling breakdown. She looked at me as if I were speaking a foreign language. She is now recovered and doing social studies. She wrote recently, 'How glad I am that I know what nervous suffering is all about! I go up to a patient now and from my own experience speak his language. What is more, he knows I understand. My suffering was indeed a privilege!'

We learn through contrast. We don't appreciate peace until we've known turmoil. After recovering from the torture of nervous illness, simple pleasures take on new meaning. Sitting at peace with friends means more than ever before. Instead of feeling guilty, nervously ill people should feel privileged because they gain understanding of an experience baffling to many and when recovered through their own efforts (as I teach them) have a special insurance for the future. Whereas, the person who has never experienced nervous illness is more vulnerable than he imagines.

The last hurdle

'I can't overcome the last hurdle of going out alone. From being unable to go to the end of my drive, I can now take a job in town, if I'm driven there. However, anxiety symptoms still come at frequent and unpredictable moments.' Of course they do. They will continue to come until he overcomes not only the last hurdle, but the first. Both hurdles are the same. Both come back to his learning how to cope with himself. Too many people say, 'I can now do this and that, but I can't do such and such.' They mean that they still can't cope with themselves when they panic or have other nervous sensations. They have learned how to cope with certain situations but this is going only part of the way toward cure.

Actually, the day that man first ventured outside his drive alone and panicked, he faced his first and, at the same time, last hurdle. That first panic held as great a challenge as he would ever meet again. In future situations there may be slight variation, but little will hold more challenge than that first panic outside his front gate. Whether he calls it first or last hurdle, it is still coping with himself, inside his drive, outside his drive or in the town centre. Recognising this and not trying to compromise by coping with one situation after another is a big step towards cure and means truly understanding agoraphobia.

This man has improved by depending on certain props and I'm not detracting from his success, but he has not yet gone through that last 1 per cent of 100 per cent acceptance, and until he does, anxiety symptoms will continue to come 'at frequent and unexpected moments', although they are not as unexpected as he thinks. He has prepared the way for them by accepting only 99 per cent. One hundred per cent acceptance is the first and last hurdle.

Why setbacks impress more than progress

Progress is difficult to estimate. You don't usually *feel* progress. You may sometimes have to convince yourself that you have made progress. True, there are moments when an agoraphobic can be elated with success, but elation is fleeting, while the apprehension that comes with setback lingers. There is no question about not feeling a setback. Setback is all feeling: dampened hope, despair and usually a return of nervous symptoms.

Also setback reminds of past suffering and even the memory of suffering can make a deep impression. I have often talked about the part memory plays, because so much nervous illness is kept alive by memory. Indeed, the memory of nervous suffering comes more acutely, more readily and lingers longer than that caused by organic illness. Nervous suffering is bewildering, relentless – an experience not easy to forget. It is important to come to terms with memory as soon as possible, so that, when it brings back the ghosts of previous suffering, you will not think immediately, 'I'm ill again! I'm back where I started!'

Memory does not haunt all who have recovered from nervous illness. I have known people recover instantly on explanation of their illness. A man wrote, 'I have been put in charge of the section at work and I am actually managing. I feel confident now that if a setback comes I shall know how to deal with it. I am armed with a technique and an understanding of what is happening. With the mystery gone, the bomb is defused.'

A husband said, almost jokingly, 'I almost wish my wife were ill again, and couldn't go shopping. That's the third hat she's bought this week. She can't pass a shop now!' On her first visit to me, he had had to lead her into my office and she had not been into a shop for two years. After explaining sensitisation to her and teaching her how to cope with panic, I pointed out that she should welcome returns of panic as an opportunity to practise coping with it. A week later, she said, 'I can't panic any more! I went to the top of the A.M.P. building [one of the tallest in Sydney] and looked over. I couldn't panic, even then!

What will happen if I can't practise?' Her cure was instantaneous.

Fear of meeting people

'I'm doing fine with agoraphobia, but I'm afraid of contacting and talking to people, especially strangers.' Fear of talking to people is another complication of emotional reaction coming to intensely and too quickly. Because of this, a sufferer feels self-conscious and vulnerable to what people may think of him. Also, he resents his attention being demanded when he thinks he must give all attention to himself, while he tries to appear normal. He is not as afraid of people as he thinks; he is afraid of his reaction to them.

This man should not be discouraged into thinking that meeting people will always be so difficult. The more he practises, of course, the better. However, at this stage, he must not grimly push himself forward. When he does meet people he should be satisfied to function to the best of his ability. Post-mortems do not help. How he manages now has little bearing on how he will manage when well. As he recovers, the curtain between him and the outside world will lift so that he will feel freed from himself and staying on guard while he talks will be no longer necessary.

It may comfort him to know that many people are shy, feel awkward, in a similar situation. Mixing and talking at ease takes practice like any other skill. However, nervous illness encourages seclusion, so nervous people have little opportunity for such practice. These people are like a crayfish that has cast its old shell and is waiting for its new, soft shell to harden. The soft shell is so vulnerable to any outside mishap. So, when this man is apprehensive about meeting people, or feels anxious while talking, he can help himself by thinking, 'It will still take time for my new shell to harden. I must not expect too much from myself at this stage!'

What's the use of making an effort?
On some days, agoraphobics struggling to move about alone, feel overcome by failure and exhausted by effort and think, 'What's the use? I'm getting nowhere. Why struggle any longer?'

Thinking 'What's the use?' is tempting at times, but it will never cure. If you feel this way and are honest with yourself, you will find that too often you added second-fear and accepted very little. I suspect also that you may have overtired yourself with your courageous but misdi-rected effort. The grim fighter is soon depleted. The cowardly custard quickly running back home is less likely to be exhausted than he who fights on.

So, first recognise your mistakes, try to see a clear pic-ture of what you should do, and make up your mind to do it the next time you go out. But don't thrash yourself by making effort if you feel overtired. What may seem im-possible one day, when overtired, can be well within your grasp the next day, if refreshed. But I mean *overtired*, not just tired. There may be few days when you don't feel tired. And don't put off making effort until you 'feel like it'. Waiting to feel like it is too big a temptation to stay sitting at home. Few agoraphobics ever feel like going out alone. For a long time there may be inertia, fear, excuses.

So turn 'What's the use?' into 'Make the effort!' when you know you are not genuinely overtired. But, make that effort the right way. Any other way is indeed, no use. And don't wait until you are encouraged by the family. A woman complained, 'My husband won't even read the book or journals, although I need his help badly. In des-peration, the other day, I thought, "Blow everyone! I'll do it myself, alone!'' I am.'

'Dr Weekes depends on us sick people having enough will power to do as she says.'

My teaching does depend on your will power to get you started. But I know you have it. It takes will power for an agoraphobic to face a journey alone and yet thousands, who, in the beginning, thought they had no will power are facing long journeys alone at this moment. I have given you the tools, and you too have the will power to use them, if you want to. *Wanting* is the key to *finding*.

Take heart. A woman from Memphis said recently on the phone, 'One of the worst aspects is getting myself up and outside my front gate. Once out, it's amazing how easy it all becomes if I do it the right way and how difficult, how exhausted I am, if I do it the wrong way. Doing it the right way sometimes seems so simple (although not always easy) that I can't help marvelling why I didn't, years ago, think of this way myself instead of being a prisoner for so long in my own home.'

To get started, first want will power determinedly; then it will be there. Determination and lack of will power are strangers. As you work the right way, you will draw less on will power and more on the joy of achievement. Good luck.

Do nothing

A man wrote asking for a list of dos and don'ts. One do alone will cure him. *Do nothing*. Simply, do nothing. In a moment of panic-crisis, when this man thinks he can't remember my teaching, all will be well if he does nothing. Doing nothing is another way of accepting. I don't mean that he should lie in bed gazing into space, literally doing nothing. He must go out and accept challenges. Second-fear is the bogey that is keeping him ill. If he does nothing in a crisis, he won't be adding second-fear, will he? So, in moments of super-panic, simply doing nothing will eventually desensitise and cure.

'If the fear is not too intense, Dr Weekes's method works well.'
However intense the fear, the method works. The writer of that letter made the old mistake of expecting immediate relief from panic *as soon as* he begins to practise acceptance and letting go. A body may be so sensitised and the pathway to panic so well prepared (the green light all the way) that no amount of letting go at a particular moment may soften a specially severe flash of panic *at that time.*

However, because of willingness to try to let go and accept panic and other nervous symptoms, the undercurrent of release from some tension that this brings, however slight, begins to desensitise and in time panic spasms come less and less severely.

Accepting all the time
A young man who had been ill for ten years wrote, 'Although I'm convinced Dr Weekes's teaching is right, I still find it difficult to truly accept *all the time* and stop adding second-fear. I now have an understanding of my illness which has given me strength. I'm initially disappointed when I have a setback and I'm not always successful at ignoring it.'

Very few accept all the time. It's possible to accept 100 per cent one moment and fail utterly the next. One woman said, 'The further apart the setbacks are the more shock they bring and the harder it is to remember quickly what I should do. It's especially hard to accept once again!'

Of course, if you could accept all the time, you would be quickly cured. However, I neither expect you to be quickly cured, nor to accept all the time. This is why I keep encouraging you and never seem impatient however long you may linger on the way to recovery. I understand how, on some days, you can accept much, on others, little, and how confused you can be by inconsistent progress. But I also know that if you take the setbacks in your stride, as time passes, you will eventually glimpse recovery, like an explorer seeing at last the promised land.

Tranquillisation

'What should one do about occasionally taking a sedative? The present day drug-scene is rather off-putting.' This man, after practising my teaching for three years, has successfully begun music studies, goes to evening classes, and has been back at work without taking a day's sick leave in three years. Setback, he says, is initially upsetting but he draws from 'the foundation of resilience' he now has.

When a patient begins to cope with himself, I encourage doing without tranquillisers. Fifty per cent of my patients recovered without ever using tranquillisers. However, the occasional tranquilliser does no harm, especially to older people. I prefer young people, after the most acute phase of their illness has passed, to lose the habit of taking tablets. Yet again, even after recovery, a person in a prolonged stressful situation (such as an impending divorce) may occasionally need the help of a sedative or tranquilliser. The doctor should know the patient and the circumstances.

The following letters illustrate different attitudes to tranquillisation. 'I feel I'm coming to terms with myself in this so difficult anxiety state. I make haste slowly; the best way. I'm fortunate in having an understanding doctor. On his instructions I'm still on tranquillisers when I feel I need them, which is not often now.'

Again, 'I have been a sufferer for ten years and have had treatment from many doctors who have been patient and kind and have given me various drugs, but these did not help. Dr Weekes's teaching has helped immensely. It is a relief to find someone who understands the terrifying experiences one goes through. *Without any tablets* I now live again. My husband and I have been on holiday and I've enjoyed this more than for many years. I'm looking forward to going to new places and only a little while ago I was afraid to leave home.'

Once more, 'Since following Dr Weekes's advice, I haven't had to take tablets regularly, except on one or two occasions. At this moment the world is a wonderful place. I can hold down a job, visit my sick husband in hospital. I even managed to cope when he was on the danger list. I've had agoraphobia since I was fifteen, I'm now thirty-four. I feel better than ever.'

Admitting you feel well

One woman wrote, 'I didn't answer your last questionnaire because things were going so well, I thought I might tempt providence if I answered it. I still have a fear of admitting I feel better because something invariably goes wrong if I do.' Any upsetting event during the early stages of recovery seem especially designed by a jinx to thwart the struggler's efforts. Fate rarely clears the way for recovery. However, the wrenches that get thrown into the works are no more than the strains of ordinary living. The person trying to recover thinks they come at the wrong time because his feeling of recovery is so new, fragile, precious.

When you feel better, don't be afraid to challenge fate by admitting it. It cheers those around you and convinces them that you are not hugging your illness. Even the most considerate member of the family may vaguely have this suspicion.

A few hours of cheerful hope from you can be respite for a harassed family. But explain that 'downs' may come again.

Prepared in this way, the downs for the family, and you, may not be quite so devastating. Have the courage to admit the good spells.

Agitation at the thought of entertaining

'I've done well with agoraphobia but my husband has to sometimes entertain clients and I can't stop getting worked up at the thought of it. I'm a rag by the time the guests arrive and want it to be over as quickly as possible.' You're not the only hostess who wants this. A non-nervously ill, middle-aged woman once said to me, 'My husband and I agree that the best moment of a dinner party is when we close the door on the last guest.' Some nervously ill people forget the strains of ordinary living, especially the strain of entertaining. They think that when cured all should be peace and roses. I wonder how many hostesses, who do their own chores, enjoy giving parties. There is always some strain: will the food be all right, are the guests going to suit each other, will the hi-fi break down as it did last time, is the noise from next door too loud? None of these induces tranquillity or helps to maintain the poise the writer of that letter envies. Of course, her agitation is based on more than worrying if the hi-fi will break down. She worries for fear she will break down.

In recovery from nervous illness, tranquillity on entertaining is one of the last achievements. It's a wise person who accepts this and is prepared to entertain to the best of her ability, even if this means trembling hands occasionally spilling coffee in the saucer.

Inability to think in a crisis

'I can believe in Dr Weekes's teaching for ordinary daily routine matters; but it's hard on special occasions to think at all, let alone remember what she says!' But my teaching shows a way through even this moment of apparent inability to think. The truth is that this woman does think – all the wrong thoughts – and it's what she thinks, not an inability to think, that makes the occasion so specially upsetting. She thinks, 'Now I really will collapse! This is *it!*'

However, I understand her. She means that at the moment when she tenses herself into super-panic, she feels paralysed with fear and my teaching then seems beyond her reach. At such a moment she must be willing *to not think*. Her feelings will gradually calm if she is prepared to stay 'paralysed in thought' and not try 'to do something about it.' She can be assured that no one can stay like this for long. Gradually the body takes over, despite fear. Eyes begin to see, ears to hear and legs to move. Nobody can sustain that flash moment of nothingness indefinitely. This apparent inability to think is only super-panic brought on by her own fear of it.

I understand that this woman is afraid, not only of not thinking, but also of what she imagines she may do in such a moment of apparent loss of control. She vaguely imagines herself going berserk, although she does not quite understand what this means. Going berserk, for her would simply mean running off in hysterics. However, becoming hysterical is quite a feat, almost an accomplishment. It takes effort to swing up into the emotional outburst hysteria demands and then perseverance to maintain it. This kind of energy can hardly be available in a moment of nothingness. She need have no fear of going berserk. I've never yet seen an agoraphobic in hysterics. As I mentioned in one of my earlier books, if, at a social gathering, an agoraphobic finally decided that he could not stay a minute longer in his seat and must go outside, he always manages to say politely 'Excuse me, please!' as he squeezes past the people beside him.

So, in a moment of crisis, if you believe you cannot think, be prepared not to think, not to remember what I say. By willingly thinking nothing (or willingly believing you are thinking nothing – there's a difference), you are as close to acceptance as could be expected in such a crisis at this particular time in your illness. Not thinking at all, *if done willingly*, will help to cure you.

Sitting quietly in public

'I'd like to know a little more about how to practise sitting quietly in public. I still can't grasp the meaning of floating. If I went queer and panicky at a social meeting, how would I cope? I can't relax and "flop" while I have to keep up appearances, can I?' When I say let your body flop during panic, I don't mean that you do this so well that you slide off your seat. I mean that you feel the sensation of flopping *inside yourself*. Loosen that tight hold on yourself and let your body sag just a little in your chair.

Sit in a chair and practise now. Imagine you are in the front row of a social gathering with no easy escape. Notice how your abdominal muscles almost immediately stiffen. Take a deep breath and let it out slowly. Relief comes best at the end of a deep breath. And as you breath out practise releasing those tight tummy muscles. It helps if you try to feel your chest sinking down into your abdomen, as if your whole body was sinking through the chair. As for appearances, the most anyone would notice would be a slight drooping of the shoulders.

If you practise inside-flopping while you panic, the

panic will not seem so searing. Slack strings cannot be twanged as forcefully as tight strings, so loosen your 'nerve strings' by simply letting your body go slack.

Cut off from the world

'I would like help about what to do when I feel momentarily cut off from the world, not there. I'm very determined to overcome this.' She will, if she does what I now teach her. Incidentally, she is still young — only sixty. She has made much progress: can now use a self-operated lift, travel in public transport, shop. She still books a seat at the end of the row at the cinema, 'just in case', but she works with fewer props.

Feeling momentarily cut off from the world, of not really being 'there' is inevitable for many nervously ill people, because their thoughts are so often *not* there; they are turned on to themselves, their feelings, the effort they are making at that moment. So the strange feeling of being only partly in the world is natural on such occasions. Once more, this is no more than one of those 'strange feelings' that may come with nervous illness at any time, even during recovery, and I have impressed on you so often not to be bluffed into being frightened by strange feelings. However horrible, bizarre, they carry no portent for the future.

A feeling of not being there is even part of the routine of recovery. So please, try to understand it and go on with the job in hand until the time eventually comes when the feeling means so little, you hardly notice it.

'A stupid old fool!'

In answer to 'What is your attitude to setback?' one woman wrote, 'After reading your book and listening to your records many times, my attitude is easier; I'm not so tense. On the days when I feel apprehensive, I hear your voice and I say to myself "You stupid old fool, be patient! Relax and it will pass as it always has. This isn't easy, but I'm not so frightened." I guess she's not the only one who has called herself a stupid old fool?'

Another answer to 'attitude to setback': 'I just don't know how I'm going to get through another bout of it!' You would be surprised to know how many she's been through since writing that letter. What alternative had she?

If some of you become as fed up as that woman and decide to give up the fight, give my teaching away, the release from trying brings some relief and for a while you may feel better. Giving up is a form of acceptance. However, the voice of conscience will soon niggle. When conscience forces you outside once more, go as resignedly as you can manage. *Take the fight out of trying.* If only I could get this message across to you, your battle would be over.

One man said, 'I get depressed with setback and frantically try to stop it escalating!' He certainly is not resigned. The 'frantically' is his undoing. How can he expect to stop nervous symptoms coming, while he is frantic? Frenzy and nervous illness share the same symptoms. With acceptance, setback will not escalate. With frantically trying to fight it, it certainly will. Fight and frenzy bring tension; tension brings more sensitisation, more symptoms (hence the escalation). Resigned acceptance bring a certain calmness which, however slight, takes the biting edge off setback.

Permanent cure

An agoraphobic woman journalist described recently in a magazine article how, by using a particular tranquilliser, she had been able to lead a normal life for the preceding six months. She praised the drug (one in common use) and added, 'I have only one bridge left to cross. My doctor says I must soon stop taking the tablets. I admit I feel apprehensive, but I'm hoping all will be well.'

I would not want a patient of mine to face the future merely hoping all would be well. This woman's cure now rests on the chance that when she stops taking the drug, she will not panic again. But she is already apprehensive and there is only slight difference between pangs of apprehension and spasms of panic. She is already sensitising herself.

For permanent cure, learning how to cope with panic is essential, because once a person has suffered from nervous illness, memory, in an unguarded moment, can bring a return of panic in many different ways, places. *And there is no drug to stop memory.* So, if this woman's memory brings a return of panic, she may too easily succumb to depending on tablets again and then later be faced with the necessity of once more doing without them. Such repetition of dependence is a poor recipe for encouraging confidence.

Surely it is obvious, that for permanent cure, you must learn how to cope with panic and other nervous sensations, so that you take your cure with you, wherever you may be.

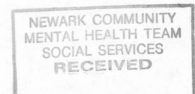

References

1. Marks, I. M., *Fears and Phobias*. London, Heinemann, 1969.

2. Weekes, C., *Self Help for Your Nerves*, London, Angus & Robertson, 1962. Published in America as *Hope and Help for Your Nerves* by Bantam Books Inc., New York, 1977.

3. – *Peace from Nervous Suffering*, London, Angus & Robertson, 1972; New York, Bantam Books Inc., 1977.

4. – *Hope and Help for Your Nerves*. An album of two cassettes available from Relaxation for Living, 29 Burwood Park Rd, Walton-on-Thames, KT12 5LH, United Kingdom; Worth Productions, PO Box 30, Neutral Bay Junction 2089, Australia.

5. – *Moving to Freedom; Going on Holiday*. Cassette. Available as above.

6. – *Good Night, Good Morning*. Cassette. Available as above.

7. – 'A Practical Treatment of Agoraphobia'. *British Medical Journal*, 1973, 2, pp. 469-71.

8. Harper, M. & Roth, 'Temporal lobe epilepsy and the phobia – anxiety – depersonalisation syndrome'. *Comparative Psychiatry*, 1962, 3, pp. 129-51.

Index

DR CLAIRE WEEKES SPEAKS

Dr Weekes gives further help on cassettes and videos for sufferers from "nerves". The cassettes are called:

Hope and Help for Your Nerves
Good Night, Good Morning
Nervous Fatigue — Understanding and Coping with It
Moving to Freedom, Going on Holiday

The cassettes are available from:

Australia
Worth Productions
PO Box 30
Neutral Bay Junction
NSW 2089

United Kingdom
Relaxation for Living
29 Burwood Park Road
Walton-on-Thames
Surrey KT12 5LH

USA
Living Growth Foundation
Box PO 48751
St Petersburg, Florida 33743
Tel: 813 345 8831

The videos are available from:

United Kingdom
Pacific Recordings
32 Woodside Drive
Cottingley, Bingley
West Yorkshire BD16 1RF

USA
Living Growth Foundation
Box PO 48751
St Petersburg, Florida 33743
Tel: 813 345 8831

Videos will be available in Australia soon.